FEMALE EJACULATION
& THE G-SPOT

"This is going to be bigger than The G-Spot... super informative, with the distinctive Sundahl style from *On Our Backs*. [Deborah Sundahl is] the only person who could write the book in this way—extremely knowledgeable and ever so fun to read. It is a revolutionary book."

DEDICATED TO the special beings

who are helping us access

the beauty and healing

that exist on the higher planes

of our human erotic landscape.

deborah sundahl

female ejaculation &
THE G-SPOT

not your mother's orgasm book!

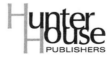

> Hunter House Inc., Publishers
> PO Box 2914
> Alameda, CA 94501-0914

Illustrations on page 28 reprinted courtesy of the Federation of Feminist Women's Health Care Centers. Illustrations on pages 32 and 33 reprinted courtesy of Milan Zaviacic. Illustration on page 56 reprinted courtesy of the Nik Douglas collection. Illustration on page 56 reprinted from *Erotique du Japon.*

LIBRARY OF CONGRESS CATALOGING-IN-PUBLICATION DATA
Sundahl, Deborah.
    Female ejaculation and the G-spot / Deborah Sundahl.— 1st ed.
    p. cm.
    Includes index
    ISBN 0-89793-380-X (pb)
    1. Women—Sexual behavior. 2. Female orgasm. 3. G spot. I. Title.

HQ29 .S86 2002
306.7'082—dc21   2002024298

PROJECT CREDITS
Cover Design and Book Production: Brian Dittmar
Developmental Editor: Laura Harger
Copy Editor: Rachel E. Bernstein
Proofreader: John David Marion
Indexer: Nancy D. Peterson
Acquisitions Editor: Jeanne Brondino
Editor: Alexandra Mummery
Editorial Assistant: Caroline R. Knapp
Publicity Coordinator: Earlita K. Chenault
Sales & Marketing Coordinator: Jo Anne Retzlaff
Customer Service Manager: Christina Sverdrup
Order Fulfillment: Lakdhon Lama
Administrator: Theresa Nelson
Computer Support: Peter Eichelberger
Publisher: Kiran S. Rana

Printed and Bound by Bang Printing, Brainerd, Minnesota

Manufactured in the United States of America

9 8 7 6 5 4 3 2 1   First Edition   03 04 05 06 07

Contents

Illustrations

Foreword

The knowledge that some women ejaculate at the moment of orgasm was, like many other important aspects of sexuality, buried by Puritanism and patriarchy. In 1978, when I first read the article "Concerning Female Ejaculation and the Female Prostate," by J. Lowndes Sevely and J. W. Bennett, in the *Journal of Sex Research*, I dismissed it as arcane and peripheral. But merely two years later, when I learned about research on the same topics by John Perry and Beverly Whipple, it became clear to me that I had, once again, been the victim of the antisexual bias of the culture in which I was raised. Female ejaculation, far from being arcane and peripheral, is an important part of some women's sexuality. Women who ejaculate should know that, and so should their partners.

Not all women ejaculate, nor do they need to do so in order to enjoy a life filled with sexual pleasure. Some women are natural ejaculators. Others have taught themselves to ejaculate. To make it a standard or a goal for all women would be foolish and destructive. What is vitally important is that women who experience ejaculation know that it is normal, that ejaculate is not urine, and that there is no need to hide their ejaculation experiences or to take measures—as some have done with the help of surgeons—to eliminate ejaculation. Because women feel, just before ejaculation, a little like they do when they need to pee, many women have been afraid to allow themselves to let go into orgasm, much less ejaculation.

We don't yet know why some women ejaculate and others do not. Nor do we know exactly the bodily source of female ejaculation, why ejaculation exists, or what evolutionary function, if any, it performs. We do know that it exists and that it gives much pleasure both to women who ejaculate and their partners, providing that the women and their partners know that ejaculation is normal and that ejaculate is not urine.

Deborah Sundahl has done us an enormous service by putting together in one book all that is known about the subject. This is not her first pioneering effort on behalf of women's sexuality, and I suspect and hope it won't be her last.

—— ALICE LADAS
coauthor and researcher
*The G-Spot and Other Discoveries
About Human Sexuality*

Santa Fe, New Mexico
April 2002

Foreword

When I started facilitating women's sexuality workshops fifteen years ago, I had never heard of "female ejaculation." The concept simply didn't exist in the public consciousness. In retrospect, I had ejaculated several times, including once in a sex film, *Deep Inside Annie Sprinkle*, in 1981. However, there was no name for what had occurred. I had no knowledge of what my body was doing, nor did my lovers, nor did adult-industry fans, nor even other women. It was just something that happened on occasion, and I didn't think much of it. The only thing I did know was that it was extremely pleasurable!

The following year, I started hearing tales of "female ejaculation" through the grapevine. I asked a group of about forty women in a workshop I was teaching if they had heard anything about it. Two women tentatively raised their hands. We shared our limited knowledge and experience with the group.

Then a wonderful video by Deborah Sundahl (a.k.a. Fanny Fatale), *How to Female Ejaculate: Find Your G-Spot*, was born to the world. It caused a sensation! Many thousands of women bought it, eagerly studied it, and shared it with their thousands of friends who all shared it with their millions of lovers. The world has never been the same!

Today, when I teach a women's sexuality workshop, the subject of female ejaculation inevitably comes up, and most everyone in the group has knowledge of it and has experienced it in one way or another. Now, we share our experiences with authority and conviction. How exciting it has been to have witnessed so much growth in the world of female sexuality in such a relatively short time. I'm not that old, and I remember when people barely knew what a clitoris was, where to find it, or what to do with it. I remember when lots of people doubted that women actually could have orgasms, and far fewer women did. I remember when "bisexual" was a rarity, and "queer" was a majorly dirty word. I remember when women weren't expected to enjoy sex at all, but to have constant "headaches." We *have* come a long way, baby!

Sexual knowledge can, and unfortunately often does, remain a sexual secret. However, when shared, the good news travels faster than a hundred monkeys learning to wash sweet potatoes. Today, women (and other genders) are freely enjoying big, woman-made, wet spots in beds around the world. Women are asking for what they want and need sexually, and are likely more satisfied than ever. There is still great need for more research. There's much more to learn and huge room for growth. It is well worth all of our efforts.

Our sexuality is not only something that can be used for the enhancement of an intimate relationship, for physical pleasure, or procreation. It can also be used for personal transformation, physical and emotional healing, self-realization, spiritual growth, and as a way to learn about all of life and death. An honest, sexually knowledgeable woman, or group of women, is a divine and extremely powerful force that not only can inspire other women, but also has the potential to contribute to the well-being of all life on earth.

You go!

> — ANNIE SPRINKLE, PH.D.
> Erotic performance artist/
> prostitute/porn star turned
> sex educator/sexologist
> San Francisco, California
> May 2002

Acknowledgments

I thank all the women who have come forward with their stories of ejaculation. Their courageous and heartfelt tales inspired me to continue with my work in the early days, when denial of female ejaculation came fast and furious from every possible avenue.

I want to thank Hunter House for being the first publishers in the country brave and farsighted enough to publish a book on the subject of female ejaculation. I am deeply grateful to the Hunter House staff: to my editors Jeanne Brondino, for her kind words and support for the topic, and Alex Mummery, for the opportunity to try new word-processing software that is a delight to use, to Kiran Rana for his care and thoughtfulness with managing the cover design, to Rachel Bernstein for her careful work as copyeditor, and to Caroline Knapp for being a delight to work with and pushing the book through the final editing stages. To Laura Harger, I owe my thanks and appreciation: Her skillful editing eye assisted me greatly in organizing the material and crafting a useful and practical book, and she was a guiding hand in this project.

To Christi Cassidy, I give my utmost thanks for her unfailing support and professional advice as I wrote the book. Her mothering made my first book-writing process considerably less nerve-racking than it would have been, and she helped minimize the many faux pas this novice writer would have made. I thank Alice Ladas and Annie Sprinkle for their kind words of support in the forewords; Suzann Gage, R.N., and the Federation of Feminist Women's Healthcare Centers for generously sharing their pioneering medical illustrations in this book; and Nik Douglas for the lengthy loan of an original photo from his erotic art collection.

Thanks to my friend Moti Melchizedek for applying her artistic talents to illustrating this book. To my partner Ed Conley, thanks for his incredible patience, first class cooking, and loving support throughout this process. To my son Aaron Schultz, thanks for being the best son a mother could have, and for encouraging me to continue my work during somber years when the struggle seemed not worth the effort.

My thanks to Grandma, Mom, Dad, and my sister and brothers, sisters-in-law and brothers-in-law, uncles, aunts, and cousins for graciously accepting the subject matter their kin and offspring desires to write about.

I express my gratitude to authors and researchers Alice Ladas, Dr. Beverly Whipple, and Dr. John Perry for their groundbreaking work that inspired me to learn all I could and teach others about female ejaculation. I also offer my thanks to Dr. Milan Zaviacic for his equally pioneering studies on the anantomical reality of female ejaculation and its source, the female prostate—his findings provided the scientific foundation for this book as well as renewed enthusiasm for and confidence in the writing of this book.

I want to thank my e-pen pals from the Internet G-spot group for their openness in sharing their experiences and opinions about female ejaculation. Most importantly, I wish to express my gratitude to my colleagues, especially those who have given their expertise and energy to my projects and/or appeared in my videos. Many of these colleagues are female sex pioneers with whom I have shared much in so many ways over the years. I have benefited from knowing and working with them, and they are fondly regarded and esteemed. They have struggled tirelessly to birth women's erotic voices. Their ideas, efforts, and willingness to put their bodies on the line at times to get the message out there allowed me to draw on their courage, creativity, and strength. They are many, varied, and admired.

Many blessings to all of you.

Preface

◆

This book on female ejaculation and the G-spot is the culmination of my professional work and personal discoveries, which began in 1984 with the first time I ejaculated. I was taken totally by surprise. I didn't realize then that the stimulation my G-spot was receiving from my partner's long, slow strokes was swelling my G-spot to the bursting point with ejaculate. Finally, fluid just erupted from my body—and all over the hardwood floor!

I put my nose in it immediately, for I had some vague sense that it wasn't pee. Indeed, it had no smell at all—or, if anything, an aroma that was rather fresh and light. Some area deep inside my womb felt nearly paralyzed with relaxation and satisfaction. The rest of my body didn't feel inclined to move much, either. I mopped up the puddle and began research on what in the world had just happened to me.

I had begun a career in women's sexuality only a year before when I'd become the copublisher of a women's erotic magazine, *On Our Backs*. I financed the magazine by working as an erotic dancer in the evenings. In the early 1980s, it was unusual for a woman to take her erotic voice seriously and to consider any public act of creative sexual self-expression, whether on stage or in a publishing office, an act of self-empowerment. But because of my college education in women's studies, through which I learned the importance of telling women's stories and uncovering the truth about women's lives, I saw a need to assert the woefully absent feminine voice in the realm of sexuality. I filled this need by discussing women's erotic lives in that groundbreaking magazine for ten years, and by presenting a proud and sex-positive attitude using my female erotic energy onstage, along with my fellow erotic artists, for the predominantly male patrons.

My budding career influenced and dovetailed with a budding and exciting time of sexual self-discovery for women. The best example of this growing public female interest in sexuality was when, only two years into publishing the magazine, I was asked to teach How to Strip for Your Lover classes. Women from all walks of life came to the class to learn how to dress up in sexy lingerie and move their bodies in ways that at that time were not as commonly seen in movies and on television as they are today (nor was the lingerie available in department stores). For the many years I taught these classes, they were always full to capacity with enthusiastic women.

My surprise experience with female ejaculation was just one of many sexual discoveries I made at the time. Erotic dancing gave me access to women who were very comfortable with their bodies, and the publishing business demanded that I obtain and explore new information on female sexuality. With all the information on female sexuality that was available at my fingertips, I soon discovered there was a name and explanation for my surprising splash on the floor.

In 1978, J. Lowndes Sevely and J. W. Bennett, Ph.D., published a report on the existence of female ejaculation and what they called "the female prostate," which they believed might be the anatomical source of female ejaculation. This caught the attention of sexologists Beverly Whipple, John Perry, and Alice and Harold Ladas, who began to study the phenomenon. They reported their findings at a now-historic 1980 meeting of the professional association, the Society for the Scientific Study of Sex, and scientific interest in female ejaculation was born. Two years later, the famous book, *The G-Spot and Other Discoveries About Human Sexuality*, by Ladas, Whipple, and Perry, brought female ejaculation into public awareness.

But curiously, public attention focused solely on the G-spot, not on ejaculation. The G-spot quickly became a sought-after prize, and a hunt ensued to discover that golden treasure located somewhere in the vast ocean of a woman's erotic recesses, for the public perceived the G-spot as a mysterious source of instant and unheard-of pleasure. The chapters of *The G-Spot* that were devoted to female ejaculation, however, were received with collective silence. It was as if female ejaculation was too unfathomable and too loaded with taboo to take seriously, or even to believe.

There was no way that I could deny what had happened to me; I could not deny the puddle on the floor. I began to experiment, to study, and to talk to other women. Many of them shared with me their first-time ejaculation stories. Though the variety of experience was vast, the one thing these stories had in common was the excitement that the women experienced the first time they ejaculated. It was obvious these were fond, unforgettable memories of a special and significant life event.

This effort culminated in my writing and producing a video, *How to Female Ejaculate: Find Your G-Spot*, in 1992. In the video, I communicated sexologists' research on female ejaculation, along with women's personal experiences, in a down-to-earth, fun, and accessible manner. The video also addressed the debate about whether the G-spot exists. I demonstrated in the video that, if one inserts a speculum into the vagina and simply turns it sideways, the G-spot is revealed in all its glory. There it is, so close it could bite you! We had been covering it up all these years in gynecologists' offices.

I took this video and toured the country for years in an effort to bring the news of female ejaculation to whoever would listen. I did workshops with women to teach them how to find their G-spots and to discuss ejaculation experiences. In some of these workshops, I passed out speculums. A woman's first look at her G-spot was invariably exciting and poignant. We saw that the size and shape of our G-spots varied, and that some were set a little farther back in the vagina than others. But the most important thing was that we saw our G-spots.

This new path to realizing the classic feminist goal of having control over our bodies spawned a period of liberating activity. A small but growing group of women experimented with ejaculation. They devoured the facts, and they experimented with technique and how far they could spray! And their partners were eager to join the adventure. It was an exciting business, and it was fun.

Many years later, I hit my forties and experienced an often painful and confusing transition from youthful playfulness to a midlife desire to examine the meaning of life and my own life's purpose. I took a break from my career in women's sexuality because my own sexuality, which had fueled so many professional discoveries, had gone dormant. I broadened my horizons into the intriguing fields of alternative medicine and spirituality. I studied herbology in the Southwest and became an herbalist. I read spiritual books voraciously. These new fields and avenues of interest eventually led me back to my sexuality, where even deeper recesses of my erotic self had begun to surface.

I learned that an entirely different, yet parallel, inquiry into female ejaculation and the G-spot was underway in the field of spiritual sex, most notably in the work of Charles and Caroline Muir, and also that of Margo Anand. Creators of Source Tantra and the Skydancing Institute, respectively, their work Westernized ancient Eastern philosophies and practices which intertwined sex with spirit, using sexual energy to enhance spiritual growth. The Muirs and Anand developed modern techniques from these ancient systems to awaken the "sacred spot" to heightened levels of pleasure. The successful workshops they have been teaching for over a decade include information on massaging the G-spot and honoring female ejaculation. They also drew from Western psychology to develop methods for sexual healing when the G-spot is unresponsive to erotic pleasure.

I had noticed, since the early days of my work in women's sexuality, that many women abruptly discontinue their explorations soon after making the decision to open up and explore their sexuality. I had often wondered about this reaction over the years. Now, learning about the Muirs' and Anand's work, it seemed to me that sexual healing might be of use to these women. I began to learn from these sexual healers and to discover Tantra and the art of sacred sex. Inspired, I wrote, directed, and produced another video in 1998, *Tantric Journey to Female Orgasm: Awaken Your G-Spot*, which explored the G-spot and female ejaculation from a healing, spiritual perspective. The video featured the first-ever demonstration of a G-spot massage, which is used to release emotional blocks caused by negative sexual events which have caused the G-spot to become numb or painful (Chapter 8 describes a G-spot massage session that I observed).

To me, learning about the Tantric path has been critical to understanding the role of the G-spot in women's emotional, physical, and spiritual lives, and this knowledge has also presented a solution to women who feel stuck in their process of sexual growth. My explorations in the realm of alternative healing and spirituality have shown me the G-spot's unique ability to enhance not only women's physical pleasure but also their intimate relationships with themselves and with others. The idea that female sexuality is not simple, but evolves and expands throughout one's lifetime, is an enticing promise. And at the heart of this idea—and at the heart of women's sexual evolution—dwells female ejaculation and its source, the G-spot.

I never could have guessed, that night when I stared in blank amazement at the puddle on the floor, that a powerful and profound tool to expand my ability to love myself and others lay behind this swirl of female waters between my feet. Once honored as sacred in ancient temples, female ejaculate has languished in oblivion in modern times. I hope this book resurrects the wonder of female ejaculation in all its mysterious aspects. Equally important, I hope it helps to spread knowledge about and interest in this issue, supporting the exciting scientific discoveries of these past two decades.

⊚ Important Note ⊚

The material in this book is intended to provide a review of resources and information related to female ejaculation and the G-spot. Every effort has been made to provide accurate and dependable information. We believe that the sensuality advice given in this book poses no risk to any healthy person. However, if you have any sexually-transmitted diseases, we recommend consulting your doctor before using this book.

The author, editors, and publishers cannot be held responsible for any error, omission, professional disagreement or outdated material and are not liable for any damage or injury or other adverse outcome of applying the information in this book. If you have questions concerning the application of the information described in this book, consult a qualified professional.

Introduction

When women brandished vibrators and burned their bras as a part of the women's rights movement during the 1960s, they were on a mission to discover their sexuality. Determined to no longer be solely vessels for men's pleasure, they first dismantled the old stereotypes of what gave women erotic pleasure. Then, they began discovering and naming for themselves their own unique pleasures. In doing so, women moved toward becoming men's true sexual equals rather than their sexual marionettes.

Having orgasms was first on the agenda. Anecdotally, approximately 60 percent of women were not experiencing orgasms. The absence of this basic human sexual response and pleasure in a majority of women needed serious attention. Women began masturbating and talking openly about doing so, and vibrators became common bedside accoutrements. Women discussed with their partners the need for more foreplay and oral sex, and they spent much of the 1970s teaching men to get used to these new erotic ideas and "demands," and learning to become more adept themselves at having orgasmic pleasure. Women discovered that fantasies were an aid to orgasm, and erotic stories sprang from women's imaginations and onto the pages of magazines and books. By the end of the decade, women's sexual voices had not only been birthed—they were growing up strong.

In the 1980s, the hunt was on for the buried treasure of the G-spot. The pop star Madonna helped make images of assertive women taking the lead sexually, with exuberant skill and pride, a cultural norm. Fantasies expanded into romantic and playful scenes acted out in the bedroom. Some women delved into the realm of leather-clad power games.

Women's sexual self-discoveries continued to simmer and boil in the 1990s, and a generation of women inherited the gains that their older sisters had made in defining women's sexuality. These young women were more public about expressing themselves sexually, and Spring Break beach parties and striptease clubs burgeoned with their freely reclaimed sexuality. Friends of all ages began to whisper rumors that women could ejaculate, and adult-industry stars appeared in adult films demonstrating this newfound feminine ability. Vibrators designed with an attachment to stimulate the G-spot emerged, and some women began to set their sights on learning how to ejaculate.

Over the past few decades, these new discoveries about women's bodies, their sexual desires, and the many ways in which they prefer to have these desires satisfied have kept publishers and editors busy and have greatly stimulated individual relationships. Much success has been achieved as a result of these changes, and the number of women who do not achieve an orgasm has dropped dramatically. Men and women have more variety in their sex lives and are generally more satisfied with their sexual relations due to the increase in intimacy that such erotic satisfaction engenders. This feverish search for greater sexual satisfaction is one that will likely continue for at least another generation or two.

One of the most remarkable and underappreciated aspects of human sexuality is its capacity to teach us about ourselves. It is a remarkable tool for expressing our emotions, fantasies, and desires, and for fuelling our imaginations and creativity. When we educate ourselves by becoming erotically literate and skillful, we can 1) make informed choices; 2) gain tolerance for those who choose a different sexual path; and 3) use this understanding to express ourselves. In fact, we are only beginning to understand all the possibilities opened up by sexuality, and all the ways it can affect us. Female ejaculation is no exception. It offers a wide-open door to sexual exploration—and the full results of its rediscovery may be many years away.

The more a person is in touch with her or his sexual needs, and has mastered healthy ways to express and satisfy them, the better off we all are.

Repressed sexual desires create havoc in individual lives and this seeps into social interactions. Like the air we breathe, yet are nearly unconscious of, a heightened awareness of human sexuality can subtly lead to greater levels of physical and mental health. Too often our sexual urges remain unconscious or are satisfied only at the most basic level. To be fully aware of the importance of human sexuality for intimacy and our overall health, we must pay more attention to how we feed, clothe, attend to, and celebrate its creative, playful, and self-educational power. The more we honor and care for this essential human energy and connection, the happier and more well adjusted we as individuals and our society will be.

What Learning about Female Ejaculation Can Do for You

Female ejaculation is inherently feminine, as well as fun and sexy. The sensation of ejaculating is freeing and erotic. But that's not all. Learning about female ejaculation and the G-spot reclaims a central, yet up to now missing, piece of women's sexual anatomy. Female ejaculation is every woman's birthright because all women are born with the anatomical ability to ejaculate.

Learning about the important part of your anatomy that creates female ejaculate will help you understand that the ejaculate is separate and distinct from urine. Traditionally, women have not been encouraged to let go and be themselves, either emotionally or physically, and the fear that they will urinate instead of ejaculate prevents many women from "letting go" when making love. Learning how to ejaculate is liberating—in any area of life. It can create or enhance a sense of personal autonomy and empowerment and may therefore also improve your overall health and happiness.

Experiencing female ejaculation and enhanced G-spot pleasure can be a gateway to learning more about one's emotions. G-spot arousal and female ejaculation not only alleviate sexual problems—loss of interest or malaise, physical and emotional pain, and decreased sexual satisfaction—but also increase the likelihood of women experiencing the satisfying intimacy that most of us desire. Because the G-spot is tied to the powerful pelvic nerve, its orgasms have emotional, cathartic characteristics. Expressing emotions opens the heart, increasing the potential for intimacy and expanding your creative abilities. What's more, the G-spot's sensitivity can be increased, and a numb or painful G-spot can be healed and awakened to greater pleasure.

The G-spot is such an important, even central, part of a woman's sex organ that it is almost ridiculous that so many women don't know about it. Imagine if men were told from an early age that they don't have a prostate. And that they don't ejaculate. And that if their penis spouts fluid, the fluid must be urine. We now have the opportunity to shed this kind of absurd misinformation about women's bodies, thanks to the work of sexologists and scientists over the past twenty years. Now, it is up to women to understand and use their sexual equipment, and to discover all the erotic sensations and sexual secrets this equipment can hold.

All women are physically capable of ejaculating. Based on scientific acknowledgement of the female prostate, which creates and expels female ejaculate, we know that all women are born with the anatomy to ejaculate, just as all women are born with arms, legs, noses, and ears. There are important reasons why some women don't ejaculate, and these primarily stem from a lack of information: You have to know that something exists before you can obtain the skills to use it. If people are consistently told they can't do something, they will eventually believe it and few will question the belief. This has undeniably been the case with female ejaculation. Women need to hear a loud, recurring chorus of "YES, YOU CAN!" about female ejaculation, and that is what this book provides. All signs indicate that all women can ejaculate—it's only a matter of learning how to do it, and after that, of choosing to do it—or not.

Women who wish to learn how to ejaculate will find information, encouragement, and guidance in this book. Reading about how some women are teaching themselves how to ejaculate and learning about the methods they use to do so can be inspiring. Knowing about cultures that viewed female ejaculation as healing and healthful also encourages a wholesome and natural view of female ejaculation. Reading about the exciting and welcome role female ejaculation plays in both women's and men's erotic lives and relationships today offers assurance to women who are uncertain about the naturalness of this ability to ejaculate that they possess.

Along with embracing this ability comes a new responsibility to practice safer sex. There are no studies documenting the transmission of HIV through female ejaculate. Therefore, I can only recommend that people weigh the risks on their own. However, if you are infected with HIV or have AIDS, it is essential that you tell your sexual partner(s) before you ejaculate with them. Since female ejaculate flows and often sprays, there is no way to contain it (as is possible with condoms for male ejaculate). So, it is best to abstain from sex if you or your partner is concerned about the transmission of HIV/AIDS.

Awakening one's ability to ejaculate and entering the deeper mysteries of G-spot orgasms opens up a new level of sexual discovery for women. It is assuredly a fun and satisfying journey, and very much in keeping with the progress women have made in discovering their sexuality over the last few decades. Female ejaculation could well be the crowning glory in this process of discovery. At the very least, it is a crucial milestone for women, and attaining it should be celebrated!

⬧ How to Use this Book ⬧

The book is divided into three parts that together provide a thorough introduction to female ejaculation: 1) the anatomy and history of female ejaculation; 2) some methods for learning how to ejaculate alone and with a partner (including helpful information for anybody who wants to assist a woman in learning how to ejaculate), and instructions for awakening the sensitivity of the G-spot; and 3) a discussion of how to embrace female ejaculation as a healthy part of sexual life and intimate relationships.

In Part I: The Phenomenon of Female Ejaculation, Chapter 1 shows how women go about learning to ejaculate in the setting of a female ejaculation workshop. Chapter 2 describes what female ejaculation is, and relates the modern scientific discoveries which now acknowledge the existence and function of female ejaculation and the G-spot. Chapter 3 takes a look at the ancient history of female ejaculation.

In Part II: Techniques for a Feminine Fountain, Chapter 4 guides readers through step-by-step explorations for assessing their readiness to ejaculate, and then teaches how to ejaculate alone and *without* an orgasm. In Chapter 5, you will learn about the nature of the G-spot orgasm, and learn how to ejaculate *with* an orgasm. Chapter 6 discusses taking female ejaculation into partnered sexual encounters, and describes sexual positions that aid ejaculation. Chapter 7 is designed specifically for men and offers helpful information on how to locate the G-spot and how to assist a woman in ejaculating; lesbians whose lovers are learning to ejaculate will also find valuable information in this chapter.

In Part III: Embracing the Feminine Spring, Chapter 8, gives important information about awakening the G-spot's sensitivity with G-spot massage. Techniques for couples are outlined in detail and a demonstration of these techniques by Tantric professionals is described. As I mentioned in the Preface, new interest in the ancient Tantric art of spiritual sex offers some intriguing methods for awakening a numb or painful G-spot, or for simply creating greater sensitivity and pleasure. A section is devoted to discussing possible impairments to G-spot pleasure due to traumatic sexual events, and suggestions are given about how to get these blocked ejaculate juices flowing again.

The last chapter, Chapter 9, provides a look at the sexual union of a man and a woman who have mastered G-spot and female ejaculation skills and are using them to increase the erotic, spiritual power of their intimate relationship. The book ends with a summation of the inherently spiritual and healthful qualities and uses of female ejaculation, and its applications, which extend far beyond simple sexual novelty.

I suggest that women first read the book alone if female ejaculation is an unknown phenomenon to them, or if they do not currently ejaculate but wish to learn. Also, if you are a man or woman who wishes your female partner to ejaculate, I believe the best approach is to read this book first by yourself. Then give the book to your partner and ask her to read it. Let her read the book alone and allow time for her to digest the information. It is important to minimize any outside pressure to ejaculate before she is truly ready, and it is essential that she feel ready before attempting the solo exercises I recommend for learning how to ejaculate. Otherwise, her ability to "let go," which is an essential factor in ejaculation, may be blocked.

If you are familiar with ejaculating but want to learn new tips to share with your partner, and you are both interested, then read the book together. There will be lots of ways to experiment and many topics for discussion will arise—both great ways to keep sexual communication and your relationship alive and sparkling.

However, if at any time you or your partner feels uncomfortable reading together, or appears to lose interest, allow that change in attitude to unfold. It may be due to sexual information overload, or to sensitive issues which can arise when new aspects of one's sexuality are being explored or deepened. The other partner can continue alone. Since skill building takes practice and individuals learn and experience things at different levels and paces, both partners will be aided by their practice when they come together again.

Although I generally refer to male and female couples in the book, lesbians will find that the suggested techniques and positions that are discussed throughout the book apply, in the majority of cases, directly to them as well.

The most useful, overall approach to using this book is to listen to your inner urges and do what you feel like doing. You can skip over the anatomy and history chapters in Part I and jump right into the exercises that begin in Part II. By all means, get down to business if that is what moves you! At some point, you may find the earlier chapters helpful for filling in some missing pieces. Read what you want to read, take breaks when you want to think about what you're reading, and allow time for the exercises and techniques to sink in. Sexuality is a unique and ever-unfolding part of every person, and this book is meant as a guide to help you learn more about your own. Let your waters flow!

PART ONE

the phenomenon *of*
FEMALE EJACULATION

CHAPTER ONE

A Peek Inside a Female Ejaculation Workshop

◆

For many years, I taught How to Strip for Your Lover classes to women from all walks of life. I enjoyed passing on to the ladies in my classes what I had learned over the years during my time on stage as an erotic dancer. These suburban housewives, career women, young urban artists, and newly single women in their fifties all shared a common bond—they had never removed an article of clothing erotically to music in their life. "Less talk and lots of practice" was my method for getting these gals moving down the road to freely and skillfully "taking it off" for their honeys.

In my classes, we spend a full three hours taking our clothes off and putting them on, taking them off and putting them on, bumping and grinding our way along the learning curve. I lead the group from a small, mirrored stage, shouting instructions over the boom of the music, encouraging the ladies to keep following along as I demonstrate the moves. I keep the enthusiasm level turned up high. This helps to disarm the feelings of nervousness, silliness, embarrassment, confusion, discouragement, or thoughts of "I like this; I must be a slut" that inevitably pop up when a woman first allows her sexual self-expression to emerge. At the end of the session, our bodies are drenched and weary, and the room is a virtual battlefield, with clothing and props strewn everywhere.

I teach that it is important to project an aura of sexual confidence and a positive attitude. I tell them a bit about striptease history and the basics of preparation: selecting music, costumes, and props. As we stumble through the moves, the women develop a sense of timing and learn how the entire piece unfolds. By the end of the session, they have an idea of their own unique style. When they walk out the door, they walk with actual experience under their garter belts, energized and happy, christened in performing the "art of the tease."

My classes on how to female ejaculate have similar characteristics. Learning to ejaculate is about basic preparation, basic moves, and, certainly, a basic sense of timing, rhythm, and length, all laced with an attitude of enthusiasm and confidence. A little knowledge of history and anatomy sets the stage. After that, it's down to the business of ejaculating.

We throw off our clothes, flop down on our towels, and make sure any "props" we want are close at hand. Students follow along with me as I call out instructions and keep things moving along with high energy, a dash of discipline, and lots of encouragement to push through any blocks and keep everyone focused. The women develop a sense of their unique timing, preferred techniques, and style. And when they leave, they've been christened with the true waters of womanhood, and there's a smile on each face and a bounce of newfound, uninhibited freedom in every step.

In this chapter, I'll take you inside a female ejaculation workshop in order to give you an overall idea of what is involved in learning how to ejaculate and how the process unfolds. In Part II of this book, all the instructions and terms used in the following description of a workshop session are explained in detail. You also can refer to the Glossary at the end of this book for a quick reference. For now, I hope that seeing how one of these workshops unfolds will show you just how accessible female ejaculation is, given the right attitude and some basic knowledge. So, get out your wet suits, girls! Let's get comfortable and have some fun!

☾ Bumping and Grinding Down the Erotic Road ☾ to Female Ejaculation

We are greeted at the door by an attractive, gracious workshop hostess, who escorts us into her spacious living room. Large pillows are thrown against the chairs and sofas that line the walls. The center of the room has been cleared. The lighting is warm, dim, and pleasant, and goodies are set out on the dining room table. The artwork on the walls depicts lovers entwined in various postures of erotic bliss. On a side table, a tiny sculptured waterfall offers soothing background sounds. Lush velvet drapes are pulled snugly over the windows, creating a feeling of security and privacy.

Ten women are assembling here, finding a comfortable area on the floor to sit, placing their bags of workshop items nearby. I've asked them to bring two thick towels, a small tarp or rubber-backed flannel sheet, lube, a mirror, a small flashlight, a favorite sex toy, a banana, and an object that symbolizes erotic self-love. The nervous laughter and friendly chatter die down as our hostess introduces me and welcomes everyone to the workshop.

I thank everyone for their courage and for the adventurous spirit that guided them to attend. I tell them a bit about my background and experience in teaching these workshops. Then it's time to discover who is here, whether they ejaculate and where they are in the process of developing that ability, or if they do not ejaculate, why they want to learn how.

The group is fairly representative of women who take these workshops. There are two single, wholesome-looking women in their late twenties and one rotund mother in her forties who already ejaculate. Two married friends in their mid-thirties and a bisexual college student are curious, moderately informed, and eager to learn. One recently divorced woman in her early fifties, slim and attractive, is blossoming into her sexuality after a long marriage that was not sexually satisfying. She is not sure where her G-spot is or if she even wants to ejaculate, but she is curious about anything that has to do with sex. A woman in her early thirties is here because her boyfriend wants her to ejaculate. Rounding out the group are a professional consultant in her forties and a successful writer in her sixties. They don't know much about ejaculating and are somewhat skeptical, but have come to see what it is all about.

After sharing some facts about female ejaculation, I give reasons why we may want to do it: It's our feminine birthright. It's something we naturally do. Sexual energy is creative—think what it means if our flow is stopped! It means we've blocked parts of our creativity. And it means there is a part of our sexuality that we haven't explored, that we don't even know exists.

I continue by outlining the evening's agenda. "Not only will we find our G-spot, but we will see it using the mirror and flashlight. We will test the strength of our pubococcygeus (PC) muscles with our fingers and with the banana and do some PC-muscles exercises with the sex toy. We will feel our G-spot and make it swell by using G-spot stimulation techniques that build ejaculate fluid. Then we will arouse ourselves to the point where we can attempt to ejaculate. No orgasm is necessary, as you can ejaculate without one! If you can't keep yourself from climaxing, however, no one will care or begrudge you that pleasure!"

"Now, everyone find a comfortable place on the floor. Lay down your tarp or rubber-backed flannel sheet and put your towels upon that." At this point, performance anxiety shifts into high gear, so the hostess steps up to the front of the group. While she removes her panties and sits demurely on her towel, I lube up a clear plastic speculum and tell the group what's next. "We are going to look at her G-spot! And after she is done, each woman will get to see hers and share what it looks like with the group, so that we can all get a sense of the G-spot's distinctiveness, placement, and variation in size." The hostess lifts her skirt. I hand her the speculum and hold the flashlight and mirror. I can feel the group holding its breath.

She inserts the speculum just as they do at the gynecologist's office or health clinic. The room is so silent you could hear a pin drop, were the waterfall not gurgling away in the background. Tension, doubt, fear, and contained curiosity hang in the air. She turns the speculum sideways. "Voila! There's the G-spot!" I exclaim. "Come and have a look-see."

The two wholesome-looking ladies crawl over immediately to get a front-row seat. Others crowd around and peer in. "Oohs" and "aahs" follow. The hostess points out her urethral opening and runs a finger around the spongy tissues that surround it. "The urethra is part of our sex organ. Its canal is surrounded with erectile tissue called the urethral sponge," I explain, and I proceed to give a general rundown on basic clitoral-sponge anatomy, including all the parts that make up this approximately four-inch-long erectile tissue network. "Located inside the portion of erectile tissue that surrounds the urethral canal is a woman's prostate gland—the G-spot! You can find its location by feeling its ridges." The hostess inserts her finger to show the location of the ridges. We watch as she pushes out with her PC muscles and the body of the G-spot moves forward, toward the outside opening of the vagina. More "oohs" and "aahs."

At this point, nerves have dramatically calmed and the women are dying to see their own G-spots. One by one, they get up on the pillow at center stage and everyone else crowds around to get a look. We see large ones and small ones. Some are flat; some protrude quite extensively into the vagina. On some you can see the ridges, and on others they're not as visible.

I pass out sandwich-sized plastic bags and tell them to peel their bananas and put them in the bags. "We are now going to assess the strength of your PC muscles. The first test will be to assess the state of tension in the vaginal entrance. To do this, moisten a finger, using the lubricant if you need to, and insert it into the vagina. Is it easy or difficult to enter?" Two women report that their vaginal openings are very relaxed. "Can you squeeze your finger snugly?" I ask them. One cannot achieve a snug fit. Three others report that their vaginal entrances are tight. "Push down on the perineal sponge (the anal portion of the erectile tissue network) and pry your vagina loose," I instruct. Women start to giggle, then collapse into long belly laughs. The three women push down on their perineal sponges. They understand that this action is applying deep pressure, as in massage, which forces a tense muscle to relax. I demonstrate a visualization and breath-relaxation exercise to relax tense PC muscles. (This exercise is explained in detail in Chapter 4.)

We use the sex toys to test further for tense or weak muscles at the opening of the vagina. The woman who can't achieve a snug fit also cannot tightly squeeze her dildo-sized sex toy. I tell her that her muscles are too lax, which may make it hard for her to ejaculate, and I demonstrate some Kegel exercises with the toys to show how to remedy this situation. (Instructions for Kegel exercises are included in Chapter 4.) For fun, I explain that healthy PC muscles can chop a banana in half, and the hostess demonstrates. The women are startled, and reluctant to try this one, but their curiosity wins out. Banana after banana receives its fate. One is perfectly chopped, and is held high in its little baggie and admired.

We then explore the inside of the vagina to locate the PC muscles and to measure their size and strength (you'll learn how to measure your own PC muscles in Chapter 4). Only one woman has what are generally regarded to be toned and fit PC muscles; two have tense, medium-size muscles; and, not surprisingly, the woman with weak PC muscles has a hard time even finding hers. "Keep your finger on the muscle, squeeze, and feel how it bulges up as the muscle contracts," I instruct. Then they try out their ability to isolate their pelvic muscles, and I go around the room and check that the women are not squeezing their abdomens and buttocks while they squeeze their PC muscles.

By this time, the ice is completely broken. Everyone has a feel for the state of her PC muscles, and knows where her G-spot is and what it looks like. I decide it's time to ask a few questions about orgasms:

"How many of you have orgasms primarily through penetration/ intercourse?" (two)

"How many have orgasms mostly through clitoral stimulation only?" (three)

"How many climax most often with simultaneous penetration and clit stimulation?" (five)

"How many ejaculate or feel that you could?" (three)

"How many can tell when your G-spot is being stimulated?" (two, tentatively)

The group's experiences with ejaculation, and with recognizing that G-spot and clitoral orgasms are distinct from each other, appear to be nominal. So, I explain that because the G-spot is tied to the powerful pelvic nerve, its orgasms have emotional, cathartic characteristics. Expressing emotions opens the heart, thereby increasing intimacy with others as well as our creative flow. Being essentially receptive, a G-spot orgasm requires relaxation, which heightens our senses, and it requires a free flow of movement in both body and voice. The orgasm has the potential to spread throughout the body. "See how ejaculation fits into this description of a G-spot orgasm: 'free-flowing, motion, sound, outburst of energy, cascading every-where.' " Women nod, appearing to grasp the gist of what I'm saying, if not the details.

"The clitoral orgasm is fueled primarily by the pudendal nerve. It is characterized by being genitally localized: It is not emotional, and it is more easily multi-orgasmic. Something interesting is going on here in the differ-ence between the two orgasms. Prior to 1970s feminism, many women were not having orgasms; two generations now have been raised on achieving orgasm with vibrators and clit stimulation. But Father Freud's theory has something to it. He said clitoral stimulation is for adolescents and that a mature woman learns to transfer her erotic sensations to the vagina." There is gasping and frowning and shaking of heads from the group.

"Learning to move from clit to vagina to have an orgasm is difficult if you have relied solely upon clitoral stimulation to climax. I haven't had any guides at all. Orgasming with my clitoris provided me with my first reli-able orgasms. When I think about it now, my clitoral orgasms fit in with my feminist assertiveness. I could characterize them as about me. My orgasm, my ability. But listen to those characteristics. They do sound adolescent. My orgasm, my ability, my way. Me. Hanging on to my tech-nique and demanding my orgasms. The orgasms were not deep and left me wanting more."

"Stimulating my clitoris, together with deep penetration, which stimu-lates the G-spot, slowly caused a blend orgasm began to develop. The erotic feeling was still centered in my clitoris, but longer, more emotional and satisfying orgasms began to occur. I languished in creative bliss afterward, and I felt satisfied. Why question that luscious level of satisfaction? But one day, emotional, sexual connection with a partner came knocking on my door. I wanted loving, embracing arousal and orgasm. Stimulating my clit was getting in my way."

There are more frowns, but now they are mixed with curiosity.

"Ejaculation requires stimulation by penetration or by manipulation of the G-spot. I ejaculate because I get great G-spot stimulation, because I am totally comfortable with sex, with being wild if I want, and because I'm comfortable emoting. My awareness of my G-spot has grown and, with that, its sensitivity has grown. I feel far more sensation in my vagina than I ever used to. I have learned to lose myself in the sensations rather than depend on a lot of stimulation to have an orgasm. It's great to feel this deepening of sensation. I am here to tell you: I believe there is something to Father Freud's theory. I believe that we have barely scratched the surface of the sensations and pleasure the G-spot can provide to us."

I could now see a few expressions that suggested they were willing to at least give it a try.

"So, we are not here just to focus on ejaculating, but to awaken the sensitivity of the G-spot. To be able to enjoy penetration far more than many of us do now. So let's start with stimulating the G-spot. Get comfortable, and have your sex toy handy." There is a brief commotion while the women lie down on their towels and rummage around for their sex toy.

"Moisten a finger, using the lube if you'd like, and let's explore the G-spot," I say as I lead the demonstration. "Do you all feel your G-spot? Feel the gutters on each side, feel the back side, feel the ridges. The ridges are very subtle, like a washboard, and you may not notice them at first, but if you stroke and rub your G-spot for a while, you will begin to feel them. Everyone feel their G-spot? Who didn't? Why? Breathe and relax. Keep looking." I pause to give the women some time to warm up to their first intimate encounter with their G-spots.

"What do you feel? Pleasure, pain, or nothing at all?" Three report that it feels good, two report no feeling at all, and two women say it feels like they need to pee and they don't like it. "We have blocked out this pleasure center, just as we have blocked out ejaculation. Rub your prostate—for that is what it is—firmly, but slowly, in small, circular motions. Relax as much as you possibly can. Do not tense up. Notice how it feels. Don't become discouraged if it doesn't feel like much or if it feels a bit uncomfortable. Just notice what you are feeling, and notice if you are not feeling anything. Squeeze and roll your G-spot around with two fingers. Feel it as if you were exploring your hand. Get to know its size and shape." I can sense the excitement of discovery growing in the room.

"Now, we can't do this cold and think we will feel anything at all. Let yourself become aroused; do whatever you need to do. Does anyone here have trouble becoming aroused? Please tell me if you do." No one says anything. If they do have trouble, they don't let on, perhaps preferring to just get through this session and get information that will help them to practice later, at home.

"Stimulating your G-spot may feel cold and unappealing at first, completely devoid of feeling. Then it may begin to feel pleasurable, but if you compare it to stimulating your clitoris, you may feel like forgetting the whole thing as ridiculous. That's okay. Keep going. This will change. Let's keep dropping into an aroused space. This initial coldness and disbelief that this could possibly be an erogenous zone will pass as you become more aroused. How are we doing?" I see that one woman has already stopped. "Stay with me," I say to her and the group in general. "It's just a block. Let's get past it. Feel your G-spot. Relax. You must relax and breathe!"

I take a deep breath to mentally and visibly relax my body and vagina, almost willing the group into a state of relaxed arousal.

"Feel those 'pee shots' of sensation down your legs? Those are what I call 'ejac rockets' and they're pelvic-nerve activated! Do you feel horny? How many of you feel like you are aroused enough that you'd like to forget the whole thing and just come your normal way? How many? Let's hear it! Okay, I need a few more of you to reach this level with me! The rest of us will wait a bit. Relax. Shut off everything around you. The lights are dim; no one is looking. Fantasize, play with your clit if you have to, but not too much. Rub your G-spot, try rubbing the outside of your urethra, or just inside the vaginal opening; you may like that. Get to that level of arousal where you truly feel so horny you'd like to just get to the business of coming." In the pause, I hear low moaning and heavy breathing.

"Good. How many of you feel your G-spot enlarging? Is it snug on your finger? Keep rubbing it." Two minutes elapse. "Are there more of you with me now at a higher level of arousal? Yes? Okay. Do you feel the ejac rockets? That's the ejaculation sensation. It feels like a pee sensation, but it is not. That is ejaculation knocking on your door. Relax, relax, relax. It will come. Feel how it shoots when you relax and don't think about it. Yes?

Okay. Now, keep your finger inside, stimulating your G-spot, and push out as if you're trying to pee. We are building ejaculate. Let's do this a few times, relaxing and stimulating between pushes. The ejac rockets come when you relax. The pushing builds the ejaculate." I wait a few minutes for them to get the hang of it and then say, "See! Once you are aroused and your G-spot is swollen, you can push as if to pee but you won't pee! Now, try to stay with me. This is how it will go. We are aroused yet relaxed, stimulating the spot, pushing out as if trying to pee, noticing ejac rockets down the legs, right? Yes? How many? Good. Good. Now we are going to ejaculate without an orgasm. Just push it out." I continue quickly to explain this surprise twist.

"Ignore everyone else but me. Listen to me. Take your finger out and push." "Ahhhh," someone squeals. "Put your finger back in now—except the one who just ejaculated; you push again, right now." Awhhhhh!" she screams again. "Rub! Rub!" I say to the others. "Push! Okay, kneel up. This is sweaty, fast business. I like to do this in the bathroom, where I can lie, sit, stand, or kneel, because things get a little frantic when you're trying to find the right position. Do not look around. Rub that spot. Now, finger out, and push! Hold it a beat." I ejaculate. "Ahhh, ahhh," someone else moans. There is a sound of water in the room, and it's not the waterfall sculpture. "Finger in, rub again, finger out. Push. Push!" "Ohhhh," the mother flops down on her wet towel, blown completely away.

"Push again; more will come. Push! It will feel like you are truly peeing now. You aren't. Push again. Who hasn't ejaculated but is close? Tell me. Shout out! Okay. Good. Hands and knees for you guys. Finger in. Sit back, stand up, or do whatever your body wants to do. Keep rubbing. Are you still aroused? Answer, please." "Yes, I am," a lusty, excited voice cries. "Keep rubbing, finger in. Keep rubbing. Finger out. Push. Hold a beat. Let go. Push. Hold a beat. Let go." "Ahhhhh, ohhh," another exclaims.

"Good!" I smile a big smile. "Now, let's smell it. Put your nose near the ejaculate and smell it. Remember the smell: We will share this later. Take the tissue, pat some up, and look closely at the color. Save it. Now, go to the bathroom and urinate. Do the pat test in there after you've urinated, and compare the two tissues."

Whew! Three hours later, the energy is high, and there is carnage in the room. Women are sprawled in every imaginable position. Towels are wet. One woman gave up long ago. Most have incredulous faces or big smiles. One is laughing like she has gone mad. The artist, who didn't give up but didn't succeed, isn't too pleased. "Do you want to keep going?" I ask her. "I want to go into the bedroom and try," she responds. I nod. "Yes. Go now if you feel like it." She picks up her towel and leaves.

I turn to the rest of the group. "Express your emotions, those of you who feel some. Let me hear them. Pound the floor in frustration, scream with delight. Let's hear it, everyone! Come on!" Coaching is tough work, but rewarding. Everyone is emotionally quite loose. One woman is sobbing. I watch her closely. Another is angry. I watch her, too. I laugh with joy with others and try to acknowledge with eye contact all who look my way. The sobbing woman is getting comfort. I throw the angry woman a pillow. "Punch it, scream," I tell her. "Come on, punch it." She lets loose. I throw another pillow at a woman with a shy grin. "Put that over your face and emote!" She does, hiding her face and giggling into the pillow, kicking her feet on the floor.

Things slowly calm down. I get up and pass around plastic bags for people's towels and toys, and I tell them there is food and hot tea in the kitchen. "Take a break. Then we'll come back and have a closing talk about what happened to everyone." I thank them for their efforts, and for being brave and uninhibited.

The women regroup and share how they feel emotionally and physically. I remind them that from now on it's easy, that they should simply keep becoming more sensitive to stimulation, to opening up, and to trying different positions. "Watch how your G-spot becomes more sensitive and full over time. Push out when you get really wild and stimulated, and just ejaculate on your lover, all over the floor, or wherever your heart desires. The biggest block to ejaculating is fear of letting go. When you have an orgasm, be sure to push out and ejaculate just after the swell of the wave of orgasm begins to lift you up."

I pass out ejaculation bowls to those who ejaculated and give a rose to those who didn't. We do an ejaculation blessing ceremony. We honor the ejaculate and the attempts to ejaculate that just took place in this room.

The women collect their things and leave. Each woman has taken a big step down her erotic road, including the two who didn't succeed. Sometimes the road is rough and scary; sometimes it's easy and exhilarating. I nod my head as I collect my things, wishing well to these new travelers who have joined me and many other women on a lifelong journey toward discovering their feminine erotic potential.

Society considers it "not okay" for women to be sexual in their own right. Despite a national media that talks about every conceivable aspect of sex, most American women over the age of forty were raised with the belief that "good girls are not sexual." Younger women, raised with the influence of cable TV's new explicitness and MTV's sexy videos, have taken the notion of "the bad girl" and made a public display of it, yet still the legacy of the good girl lingers, and it inhibits most women's ability to let go and enjoy.

Men's biggest sexual complaint about women is that women often cannot let go during lovemaking, and there is something to this. It simply has not been okay for women to let go and be themselves sexually, and female ejaculation shows us why in a profound way. If we let go, we'll gush all over our partner's face, chest, thighs, cock, and the bed and pillows, too! Not very ladylike, is it?

Ejaculation is real, it's fun, it's healing to our sexual psyches, and it's very female. This peek into an ejaculation workshop has touched upon many techniques and concepts that will be explained in Part II of this book. If you can't wait to learn how to ejaculate, turn to that section now and get started. Otherwise, the next chapter will provide a helpful introduction to the G-spot and the anatomy involved in ejaculation.

What *Is* Female Ejaculation?

◆

Pauline had not known about female ejaculation until she met a new lover who found her G-spot. She didn't care for the sensation at first; sometimes she felt like she had to pee when he touched it, and she asked him to stop. This stressed their lovemaking sessions until one night she found the sensation deeply pleasing and had a great orgasm. She noticed more than the usual wetness, but thought it was just his incredible skill in making her feel sensations she didn't know she could feel. She gradually became accustomed to his techniques, and one day he declared that she had produced a jet of liquid that almost hit him in the face!

She thought he was a bit crazy, and after that she noticed that she held back her sexual enthusiasm. But again, in time, she allowed herself to let go into the delicious pleasure. Then one day it happened—she ejaculated and felt the warm jet stream that her boyfriend had told her had poured out of her. Though at first she felt repulsion, she also noticed a sensation of deep relaxation. After that, it became harder to not let go, and her ejaculations became more frequent as he assured her it was normal and not urine and that he liked it.

Female ejaculation is a powerful, beautiful, healthful, and rather mysterious sexual response that comes naturally to female bodies. Once understood, its joys are many and varied, and can go deep into the heart of what it means to be female. To own the mysteries of female ejaculation requires a little faith, and for some women, a fair amount of work, but the amount of self-empowerment gained from learning its secrets makes it worthwhile.

The puzzle of female ejaculation and the G-spot began to be pieced together in the early 1980s by diverse groups of American investigators. Three groundbreaking studies brought female ejaculation into public awareness. The first, by Josephine Lowndes Sevely, was an extensive academic inquiry into its scientific past. The study revealed that female ejaculation had been known and discussed since the seventeenth century, and that its source, the female prostate, had been examined and documented. In a second study, the Federation for Feminist Women's Health Care Centers zeroed in on the clitoris and discovered that a large portion of it is hidden inside the body. Finally, in a third study, sexologists Ladas, Whipple, and Perry identified a sensitive area in the vagina that seemed to trigger female ejaculation, and they named the area "the G-spot" (after the German researcher Ernst Gräfenberg). They also identified its muscle and nerve support, and discovered it can produce its own unique type of orgasm.

Further innovative investigations into female ejaculation were done in Europe. A German academic study led by Dr. Karl Stifter concerning the cultural history of female ejaculation revealed that it was known and honored in other parts of the world. This study also documented the chemical analysis of female ejaculate. Studies in Spain by Dr. Francisco Santamaria Cabello suggested the possibility that *all* women ejaculate, though many do it "retrograde," into the bladder. The most significant study, by Dr. Milan Zaviacic of Slovakia, put to rest the debate over the existence of the G-spot and female ejaculation. It determined that the G-spot is the female prostate and it thoroughly examined its structure and the ejaculate fluid down to the cellular level, unearthing the role of the female prostate in hormone production, as well as the role that female ejaculation may play in fertility. (Turn to the section called, "All About the G-Spot," later in this chapter, for more on the Slovakian research.)

These discoveries produced a dramatic shift from the previous century's views on the female sex organ and its function and behavior, and began a process of sexual discovery and recovery of remarkable proportions for women. The general malaise women had traditionally experienced about their role in society—aptly defined in 1963 as the "problem without a name" by Betty Friedan in *The Feminine Mystique* and that kicked off the feminist movement—may have been due in part to the nearly universal ignorance of this central part of women's sexual anatomy. The benefits that arise from acknowledging all of women's sexual anatomy as functional and powerful include an increase in women's self-esteem and a powerful shift in their identity. This chapter will help both men and women understand the full structure and capabilities of a woman's sexual pleasure center.

⊚ Many Women Ejaculate—But Some ⊚ Don't Know It

Mary Beth was very concerned over this growing feeling that something was wrong with her bladder. First, there was the incident in bed with John. There was a big wet spot after they made love, and she was still mortified over this. Then, a few days later, she began to feel uncomfortable in her urethra, a very mild burning sensation, but it was persistent and wouldn't go away. Not long after that, she felt pain in her vagina when John first entered her to make love. She was wet and interested enough, so it wasn't that. The pain persisted through their lovemaking and ended up killing her enthusiasm. She noticed she was rubbing her abdomen and just feeling generally irritable and frustrated.

A few months earlier, a friend had asked her if she had heard of female ejaculation. The question shocked her, but she forgot about it. Now it kept coming to her mind. Finally, she looked in the library for some books on the subject, but found nothing there or in her favorite bookstore. Not knowing what to do, she decided to go see her doctor, thinking that perhaps she had an infection or was pregnant.

When the tests came back negative, the doctor prescribed a muscle relaxant and told her if she wasn't better in two weeks, they could do further tests to look for blockages in her urinary tract. To her relief, she began to feel better. Her symptoms disappeared and gradually her sexual interest returned. She shrugged the matter off as nerves or some unusual incident.

Women emit ejaculate fluid through the urethra when aroused and/or during orgasm. Those who have experienced it often describe it as "gushing" from the body. Until recently, very little public information existed about the phenomenon. Therefore, many women who did ejaculate were quiet about it, or mistook it for urination.

Women can ejaculate many times during a lovemaking session. Quite frequently, the amounts of ejaculate emitted increase during the session if the G-spot continues to be stimulated. Quantity can also increase over time as a woman develops a stronger sense of her G-spot and becomes comfortable letting the ejaculate flow freely.

The quantity of ejaculate varies from woman to woman, and there are many factors influencing it. These include where a woman is at in her menstrual cycle, the amount of stimulation her prostate/G-spot is receiving, her feelings about her sexual encounter, her experience and comfort level with ejaculating, the strength of her pelvic muscles, the method of arousal and type of orgasm, and whether there is something in her vagina, like a penis or dildo.

The question is often asked, "Why do some women ejaculate and others not?" I think that all—or most—women ejaculate, but not all are aware of it. They may mistake the fluid for urine or vaginal lubrication, and some may even believe they have urinary stress incontinence. Or women may control their ejaculate by unconsciously forcing it "retrograde," pushing it back into the bladder rather than out through the urethra.

Other women actually may not ejaculate because of physical or emotional reasons, despite being born with the anatomy to do so. These factors are discussed in more detail in Chapter 8. Some women don't ejaculate because of surgery that has damaged the G-spot/prostate; others because their PC muscles may be too weak to eject the ejaculate (the section "The Pelvic Muscles that Assist Female Ejaculation," later in this chapter, explains how simple exercises can remedy this). In addition, some women may be having clitoral orgasms that do not stimulate the pelvic nerve, which in turn does not stimulate the PC muscles to contract and expel the ejaculate (there's more information on these nerves in "The G-Spot Nerve" section, later in this chapter).

A reason many women produce only tiny amounts of ejaculate may be that the female prostate is conditioned to produce less ejaculate when women unconsciously control its release by clamping down on the sensation of "needing to pee." This almost instinctual, learned behavior causes overly tense PC muscles in some women and weak ones in others, and it causes some women to avoid sexual arousal altogether because they do not want to feel that urge to urinate (although, during lovemaking, the sensation of needing to pee is usually the urge to ejaculate).

A fascinating study, conducted in 1997 in Spain by psychologist and sexologist Dr. Francisco Santamaria Cabello, suggests that many women, when sexually aroused, ejaculate retrograde, into the bladder. Dr. Cabello tested the contents of the bladder in twenty-four women for prostate specific antigen (PSA)—the ejaculate identifier—before and after orgasm. Although only three out of the twenty-four women who were tested ejaculated, 75 percent of the non-ejaculating women had urine samples that had a higher percentage of PSA than had been present in their pre-orgasm urine samples. These results led Dr. Cabello to assert that women are experiencing "retrograde ejaculation," because the ejaculate fluid is being released into the bladder rather than being expelled. Some researchers have speculated retrograde ejaculation may be a cause of bladder infections in women, as it is in men.

Are you surprised to hear that ejaculation can be controlled and diverted in this way? Most public information supports the erroneous belief that ejaculation is not controllable and that only men ejaculate. But the reality is that both men and women can control whether or not they ejaculate, and both men and women can ejaculate with or without an orgasm. This ability to choose whether to ejaculate or not has been mastered by many males today and throughout history, and in some cases it is and was a cultural norm. Women will discover it is possible to ejaculate without having an orgasm, sometimes many times in a lovemaking session.

Making the choice to ejaculate or not is important for a woman's sense of personal empowerment. Choosing *to* ejaculate gives a woman freedom to use the anatomical ability she was born with in order to increase her sexual pleasure and health—and, as we shall see in the following chapters, the pleasure and health of her partner. Choosing *not to* ejaculate allows women to consciously and thoughtfully delay the experience or decline it altogether.

When women begin to investigate ejaculation for themselves, they may realize that they have been ejaculating in the past but haven't noticed it. This is because ejaculation usually occurs just as a woman begins to orgasm, which can override the sensation of ejaculating. In general, ejaculation does not make a woman's orgasm feel fuller and more satisfying; rather, it often provides a feeling of relief to the pelvic area.

ⓖ An Expanded View of a ⓔ Woman's Sex Organ

The familiar little nub fondly known as the clitoris is actually just the exposed part of the precious gem that winds much deeper into a woman's body. In 1981, the Federation of Feminist Women's Health Care Centers published a groundbreaking book titled *A New View of a Woman's Body*, which mapped an extensive network of erectile tissue that had not been covered in medical textbooks. Suzann Gage, a registered nurse, drew illustrations of the network to expose this buried treasure and declared the product "a new view of a woman's clitoris."

This network of spongy tissue fills with blood and enlarges when a woman is sexually stimulated. Aside from its well-known and well-documented parts—the glans, shaft, and legs—the Federation identified and named its previously undiscovered parts—a portion that surrounds the urethra (the urethral sponge); a portion that lies underneath the labia (the bulb); and a portion of less dense erectile tissue that lies between the vagina and the anus (the perineal sponge). The illustrations on the following page show a side view of this "new view of the clitoris" in both a relaxed and an aroused state.

The Federation's work wasn't easy. While writing the book, researchers literally found empty spaces where women's genitalia should have been detailed and discussed in both American and European anatomical textbooks. The penis and surrounding area had been thoroughly dissected and documented, but in most cases female genitals had been left *blank*.

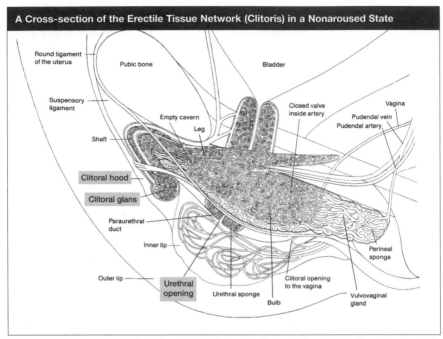

A Cross-section of the Erectile Tissue Network (Clitoris) in a Nonaroused State

Round ligament of the uterus
Pubic bone
Bladder
Suspensory ligament
Empty cavern
Closed valve inside artery
Vagina
Pudendal vein
Pudendal artery
Leg
Shaft
Clitoral hood
Clitoral glans
Paraurethral duct
Inner lip
Perineal sponge
Outer lip
Urethral opening
Urethral sponge
Clitoral opening to the vagina
Bulb
Vulvovaginal gland

Reprinted with permission from The Federation of Feminist Women's Health Care Centers. Illustrator Suzann Gage, RNCNP

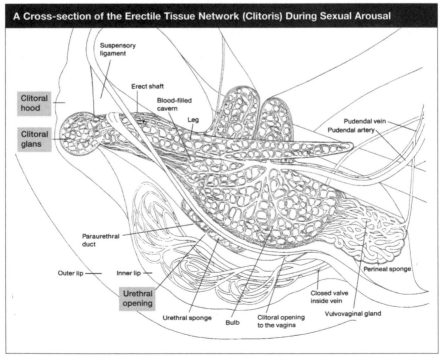

A Cross-section of the Erectile Tissue Network (Clitoris) During Sexual Arousal

Suspensory ligament
Erect shaft
Clitoral hood
Blood-filled cavern
Leg
Clitoral glans
Pudendal vein
Pudendal artery
Paraurethral duct
Outer lip
Inner lip
Perineal sponge
Urethral opening
Closed valve inside vein
Urethral sponge
Bulb
Clitoral opening to the vagina
Vulvovaginal gland

Reprinted with permission from The Federation of Feminist Women's Health Care Centers. Illustrator Suzann Gage, RNCNP

Meanwhile, Josephine Lowndes Sevely, Ph.D., published her extensive, ten-year, Harvard University–funded study in her book, *Eve's Secrets*, in 1986. Sevely reorganized and renamed the parts of the expanded view of a woman's clitoris and included the female prostate in her reorganization. Using the standard medical tradition of giving the same name to the male and female parts of the body, she created a new view of a woman's sex organ by categorizing the extensive clitoral erectile tissue network, the female prostate, the urethra, and vagina as interconnected elements of a woman's sex organ. The outcome was a complete and fully functional, medically identified female sex organ that is similar in size, structure, and function to the penis.

In addition to this anatomical reorganization, Sevely extensively researched the history of female ejaculation. She traced scientific documentation of its existence back to ancient Greek philosophers and scientists, as discussed in the next chapter, "The Ancient Herstory of Female Ejaculation." She also documented fourteen anatomical studies on the female prostate by Western scientists from de Graaf, who "discovered" the female prostate in 1672, to Gräfenberg.

The best-known of these studies, may be the 1880 study by physician Dr. Alexander Skene, who discovered two glands in the urethra that emit prostatic fluid. Though he noted their similarities to the male prostate, he thought they had no functional purpose, and therefore considered them a vestigal version (no longer fully functional, developed, or useful) of the male prostate. His primary interest was in noting that they became clogged and in explaining how to drain them. This view of the Skene's glands (a term for the female prostate that has sometimes been used in the past) as nonfunctional has contributed to the medical profession's stance that female ejaculation doesn't exist.

Today, things have changed. Medical and health-care students are receiving education in this new view of the clitoris. When a registered nurse, currently in medical school in New York, had the opportunity to witness a clitoral dissection on a cadaver, she was surprised by what she saw:

> When they cut open the clitoris, we saw it went much farther inside the body. I was awed. I realized I had only been aware of the tip of an iceberg. I immediately felt a much greater respect for what I thought was a tiny area of pleasure.

⟳ Where Female Ejaculate Comes From ⟲

Let's take a journey through this newly comprehended sex organ, to see how and where female ejaculation takes place. We'll begin with the production of ejaculate in the prostate, look at its chemical composition, and then see the role the G-spot plays in initiating ejaculation.

In men, the prostate is a large, chestnut-shaped organ that surrounds the urethra at its base, and it contains glands and ducts that emit ejaculate fluid. Like the male prostate, the female prostate has glands that create ejaculate fluid and ducts that expel it into the urethral canal. However, the female prostate is much smaller and more elongated, and is embedded in the wall of the urethra. In most women, it is located near the urethra, near the opening of the urethral canal to the outside of the body. (See illustration at the top of page 28.) It typically has about forty glands and ducts—up to three times the number found on the male prostate.

After the ejaculate is expelled from the female prostate into the urethral canal, it can flow in two directions: *out* to the urethral opening (visible/noticeable ejaculation), or *in* to the bladder (retrograde ejaculation). When the former is the case, female ejaculation commonly has been mistaken for urination because urine is all that women are expected to expel through their urethra. But urine, which contains bodily wastes, is excreted by the kidneys and accumulates in the bladder. Female ejaculate, in contrast, carries no wastes and is created in the female prostate. For women as for men, both urine and ejaculate are excreted through the urethra, despite the fact that they are distinct fluids. Scientists have measured the quantity of female ejaculate at between an eighth of a cup to one cup. However, it is not uncommon for a woman to ejaculate a far greater quantity of liquid, up to a cup and a half, in one lovemaking session—usually with prolonged stimulation and in more than one ejaculation.

In 1672, Dutch anatomist Regnier de Graaf discussed and sketched the female "prostatae," noting many ejaculatory ducts. Although de Graaf was the first to recognize the prostate as the ejaculatory source in women, it was Slovakian doctor Milan Zaviacic's extensive multidisciplinary studies on the female prostate during the past twenty years that earned it recognition as a fully functioning female organ. The medical term—female prostate—is rapidly being accepted by the medical establishment. At its 2001 meeting in Orlando, Florida, the Federative International Committee on Anatomical Terminology agreed to support use of the term "female prostate" in its journal *Histology Terminology.*

Dr. Zaviacic, a professor of pathology and forensic medicine at the Comenius University of Bratislava, Slovakia, conducted his extensive studies on the female prostate from 1982 to 1999. Dozens of full-color photos of the cellular structure of the female prostate from Dr. Zaviacic's research are included in his monograph (research book), *The Human Female Prostate: From Vestigial Skene's Paraurethral Glands and Ducts to Woman's Functional Prostate,* published in 1999. In his book, he confirms that the female prostate is a functional genitourinary organ with a specific structure, function, and pathology. "Compared to the male counterpart, the female prostate (has) a similar structure, expression of prostate markers (and) enzyme equipment...." Dr. Zaviacic also determined that the female prostate has two functions: exocrine (production of prostatic fluid—the female ejaculate) and neuroendocrine (production of hormones).

The primary function of the female prostate is to manufacture, store, and emit female ejaculate. Its secondary function is to produce hormones (the prostate's ducts are richly lined with neuroendocrine cells, which produce hormonal peptides). The range of hormonal properties of the androgen-dependent male prostate is well known, but in women only the production of serotonin by the female prostate has been established. Further research may also show that the female prostate produces estrogen and perhaps even plays a central role in a woman's neuroendocrine (hormonal) system.

◉ Types of Female Prostates ◉

In 1948, gynecologist Dr. J. W. Huffman created a mold of the female prostate from an autopsy of a woman. He discovered thirty-one ducts that empty into the urethral canal, most of them emptying into the front third. The illustration on the next page shows his model of what were called at that time the "paraurethral glands." This model is still used to represent the most common shape and location of the female prostate.

Dr. Zaviacic estimates that almost 70 percent of women have this "ramp-shaped" prostate, which Huffman modeled in 1948. Called the "meatus" type, the thickest part of the "ramp" (prostatic tissue) is located nearest the urethra. Fifteen percent of women have a prostate called the "posterior type." It is also "ramp-shaped," but the thickest part of the

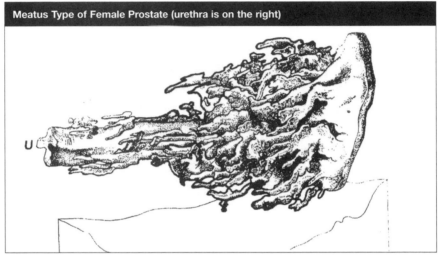

Meatus Type of Female Prostate (urethra is on the right)

Wax model of female urethra with its paraurethral (prostate) ducts and glands, Huffman 1948. Reprinted from Milan Zaviacic's book *The Human Female Prostate*, 1999

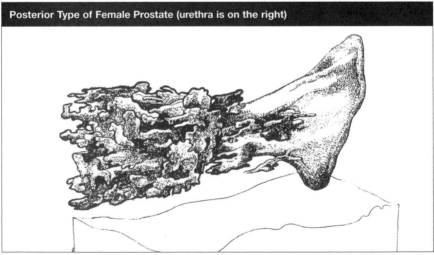

Posterior Type of Female Prostate (urethra is on the right)

Huffman, 1948. Reprinted from Milan Zaviacic's book *The Human Female Prostate*, 1999

"ramp" is located near the back of the urethral canal, nearest the bladder. In all, over three-quarters of women have these types of "ramp-shaped" female prostates.

There are two other types of female prostates that are more rare. One is called a "middle prostate," and 7 percent of women have this kind, in which prostatic glands and ducts are distributed along the length of the urethral canal, with a smaller concentration in the middle. It is also described as "dumbbell shaped." Before Zaviacic's extensive studies on the female prostate, this type of female prostate had been considered the most common. This may be one reason why people have a difficult time finding the G-spot—they are looking *too far back* in the vagina and missing the location of the most common (meatus) prostate, which is *just inside* the vagina, near the urethra, or *not far back enough*, which is where the posterior prostate can best be felt.

The other rare type of female prostate, called a "rudimentary prostate," is found in 8 percent of women. It has a scarcity of glands and ducts. Even so, in *all* cases of the rudimentary prostate, at least one or a few small prostatic glands and ducts occur. Dr. Zaviacic states that it is the female prostate's close proximity to the vagina that "enables mechanical expulsion

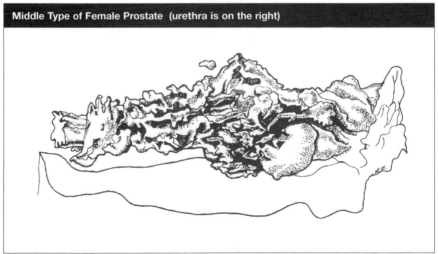

Middle Type of Female Prostate (urethra is on the right)

Huffman, 1948. Reprinted from Milan Zaviacic's book *The Human Female Prostate*, 1999 of the contents of the glands and ducts of the female prostate by pressure of the penis during penocoital friction or by contractions of the muscles around the urethra during orgasm." (We will learn how to manually create female ejaculate and expel it with fingers and a sex toy in the next chapter.) Small amounts of female ejaculate can also be expelled during sexual excitement, during physical activity, and while eliminating bodily wastes.

What *Is* Female Ejaculate?

Female ejaculate is a clear liquid. Its consistency is akin to that of very light lubricant, but it is watery rather than slick. It is not the same as vaginal lubrication or urine. Only a tiny and usually unnoticed portion of female ejaculate is creamy and white like male ejaculate, even though both women's and men's ejaculate is prostatic fluid (that is, both are created by the prostate). The taste and smell of ejaculate appear to vary with the menstrual cycle. At times it can taste and smell salty and somewhat strong, and at other times, fresh and light with an earthy, "forest floor" aroma. Sometimes the ejaculate has no smell or taste at all, or it may have the faint smell and taste of urine. Men and women's ejaculates are similar in chemical makeup, though of course women's ejaculate does not contain semen. Female ejaculate is predominantly prostatic fluid mixed with glucose and trace amounts of urine. Currently, scientists use PSA (prostate specific antigen) as a marker to identify female ejaculate.

Dr. Zaviacic's research indicated that tiny amounts of ejaculate continually seep from the female prostate into the vagina. Before the discovery of the female prostate, it was thought that only men produce PSA. Therefore, PSA has been used in tests for rape. This information that female ejaculate is usually present in trace amounts in the vast majority of, if not all, women, now calls that forensic practice into question.

Dr. Shannon Bell, assistant professor of political science at York University, Toronto, authored and produced in 1991 a feminist art video about female ejaculation, and she currently teaches female ejaculation workshops. She tested the quantity and chemical makeup of her ejaculate and reported the results in her paper "Liquid Fire," published in the feminist erotica anthology *Jane Sexes It Up* (2002). (The bibliography contains an excellent list of work of other women inspired by the publication of discoveries about the G-spot in 1982.) To conduct this experiment, she ejaculated four times in one session into a bowl and collected three-quarters of a cup of ejaculate. She describes how she tested the fluid:

> . . . poured what I could get into a test tube, capped it off and (went) to see. . . my doctor at the neighborhood health clinic who agreed just this once to test my ejaculatory fluid. In order not to disturb the lab, he put both ejaculate and urine through as separate urine samples. Sure enough: my test replicated the sexology lab tests: ejaculate has a higher pH, more gravity, less urea and less creatinine.

With the knowledge we now have of the important place of the female prostate in the woman's sexual anatomy and its analogy to the male prostate, it is not surprising that a biological use has been discovered for female ejaculate. Since the urethral canal's floor is the vagina's roof—the vagina and urethra virtually share a wall—the glucose in female ejaculate gets absorbed into the vagina. Glucose creates a supportive environment for sperm on its way to fertilization. In this way, the glucose in female ejaculate adds to the glucose in male ejaculate to create a fertile environment for sperm. Female ejaculate may thus play an unrecognized but supportive role in reproduction.

⊚ The G-Spot's Role in Female Ejaculation ⊚

We have seen that ejaculate is produced in the female prostate. The G-spot is defined as both the prostate and a network of erectile tissue similar to that found in a male penis. This same erectile tissue network extends, as we stated earlier, beyond the G-spot to include the clitoris, the clitoral legs, an area located near the anus (perineal sponge), and an area that lies underneath the vulva (urethral sponge).

When stimulated, the G-spot's erectile tissue engorges with blood and becomes enlarged. This tissue surrounds the female prostate and much of the urethral canal. When the G-spot is aroused and swollen—in other words, when its erectile tissue is filled with blood and its prostate glands are full of ejaculate—it can easily be felt through the vaginal wall. Therefore, the G-spot is not merely a "spot" on the wall of the vagina. Rather, it is an organ one can feel and stimulate *through* the vaginal wall.

The area on the vaginal wall through which one can feel the G-spot is lightly ridged. An easy way for a woman to find her G-spot is to insert a finger one to one and one-half inches inside her vagina and push it up toward the urethra, where she will feel the subtle ridges. (A women can also ask her partner to sit facing her between her legs and insert his or her finger into her vagina. This can help her feel her G-spot, and is a great way for her partner to discover its location.)

A male psychologist, communicating via an Internet G-spot chat group, described to me his experience with his partner's G-spot:

> With digital stimulation of my love's G-spot, the glands become quite
> swollen and distended. The G-spot becomes irregular and 'lumpy,'
> as if there were tiny little peas under the surface of the vaginal roof.
> I am fairly certain that these nodules are the distended lobes of
> the prostate glands.

The G-spot varies in size from woman to woman, just as vulvas vary from woman to woman. Some G-spots are small and dainty and, when stimulated, protrude rather discreetly into the vagina. On the other end of the spectrum, some are quite large and robust and, when stimulated, protrude significantly into the vagina.

A common complaint from women and men is that they cannot "find" the G-spot. This is because they are usually looking for something that triggers instant, orgasmlike sensations. In truth, the G-spot varies dramatically in sensitivity among women, from nearly numb to highly sensitive. However, much like a man's prostate, the natural state of a woman's G-spot is highly sensitive. There are many reasons why the G-spot might lack sensitivity, and many ways to increase its sensitivity. (Chapter 8, "Heal Your G-Spot," discusses why the G-spot might not be sensitive, and gives ways to heighten its responsiveness.)

Have you always believed that the clitoris was the source of women's orgasms? This is what most of us have been taught. But the G-spot is capable of triggering deep and pleasurable orgasms, too. In fact, the G-spot, not the clitoris, is center stage as the area of a woman's genitals in which she can experience the greatest and most diverse amount of erotic pleasure. This view contradicts the prevailing notions of the past century, which were that the vagina does not have enough nerve endings to create an orgasm, and therefore that a woman's central orgasmic response is located in the clitoris. However, the G-spot, like the clitoris, has its own nerve supply, one that is stimulated primarily *through the vagina.* Surprised?

The clitoris is stimulated by the pudendal nerve. The G-spot is stimulated by the pelvic nerve, one of the most powerful nerves in the body. Each nerve creates unique sensations of arousal and orgasm. Therefore, it is possible to have two different and distinct types of orgasms, or to blend the two, depending on where a woman is being stimulated. (The section "Orgasms and Female Ejaculation" later in this chapter provides more information about the different types of orgasm.)

Below is an illustration of the erectile tissue network overlaid on the most common type of female prostate. Here, finally, is the most complete picture of the G-spot.

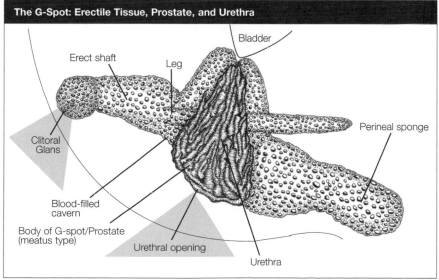

The G-Spot: Erectile Tissue, Prostate, and Urethra

Bladder
Erect shaft
Leg
Clitoral Glans
Perineal sponge
Blood-filled cavern
Body of G-spot/Prostate (meatus type)
Urethral opening
Urethra

Moti Melchizedek

Scientists have answered nearly all the unknowns about the female prostate and female ejaculate. We now understand that the G-spot—the female prostate and its erectile tissue—is a crucial part of the woman's functioning, healthy, and whole sex organ, and that a woman's clitoris, as erectile tissue, is much more extensive than originally thought. For more than four hundred years, these organs have been scientifically considered to be fragmented and/or nonexistent. As we shall learn in the next section on the PC muscles, these attitudes have jeopardized women's physical safety with serious threats to their genital and reproductive health. However, relief from damaging misinformation on the female genitourinary system is now on the way.

~ The Feminine Fountain ~

Josephine Lowndes Sevely's book, *Eve's Secrets*, offers the following descriptions of female ejaculation, garnered from experienced scientists and doctors dating back to antiquity, attesting to its authenticity, character, and beauty (as well as its effect on the recipient!):

"the movement of which excites a titillating and pleasant longing"
— *Galen (A.D. 200)*

"in libidinous women, often rushes out at the sight of a handsome man . . . a pungency and saltiness that lubricates the sexual parts"
— *anatomist Regnier de Graaf (1672)*

"being emitted as a jet, which is thrown some distance"
— *psychologist Havelock Ellis (1937)*

"clear as glass, tenacious and persistent, without being sticky"
— *gynecologist Robert Dickenson (1949)*

"out of the urethra in gushes"— *urologist Ernest Gräfenberg (1950)*

"a circular shower of jets" (when a woman is standing up)
— *urologist Kermit E. Krantz (1950)*

"two fine, angular intermittent jets" (when a woman is lying down)
— *Krantz (1950)*

✪ Pelvic Muscles that Assist Female Ejaculation ✪

In 1982, Alice Ladas, Beverly Whipple, and John Perry, authors of the famous book, *The G-Spot*, were well acquainted with the work of Gräfenberg and Sevely and, therefore, well aware of the prostate characteristics of the G-spot. They went on to not only give a rapidly adopted, popular name to this unrecognized yet crucial piece of female sexual anatomy but to identify its muscles and nerves, as well as the distinctive type of orgasm associated with it. Their book brought the G-spot and female ejaculation to public attention, and for twenty years it served as the most influential work ever produced on the subject. They also did pioneering work related to the muscles that support women's sexual response and, specifically, female ejaculation.

The illustration below shows the muscles that support the clitoral network of erectile tissue and the female prostate (as well as other organs of the reproductive area). They are called the pubococcygeus (pronounced "pew bo cox uh gee us"), or for short, the PC muscles. Fitness of these muscles is important for lubrication, arousal, and the ability to orgasm and to ejaculate.

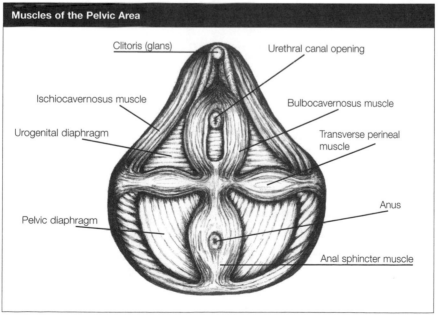

Muscles of the Pelvic Area

Clitoris (glans)
Urethral canal opening
Ischiocavernosus muscle
Bulbocavernosus muscle
Urogenital diaphragm
Transverse perineal muscle
Anus
Pelvic diaphragm
Anal sphincter muscle

Moti Melchizedek

Dr. Arnold Kegel, an obstetrician/gynecologist, was concerned about the large numbers of women who had urinary stress incontinence. In 1947, he invented an instrument called the Kegel Perineometer to give women feedback as they exercised and strengthened their pelvic muscles. A woman inserts the device into her vagina, squeezes her pelvic muscles, and watches on the dial as the gauge calibrates the strength of her contractions. This also allows her to see improvement in strength and duration, and helps her isolate and learn to use this muscle group. These PC muscle exercises are frequently referred to as "Kegel exercises." (Chapter 4 contains a detailed description of how to perform these exercises without a perineometer.)

Kegel was successful at eliminating incontinence in 93 percent of his patients. He made his biofeedback machine, with the help of his wife, on his kitchen table and offered it for sale for at-home use for a mere $40 until his death in the mid-1970s. Dr. John Perry bestows on Dr. Arnold Kegel the title "Father of Bioenergetics" because of his machine and his method. Dr. Kegel treated more than three thousand women from his suburban Los Angeles office, and wrote and published many papers on his techniques, which nonetheless languished until 1975. Some doctors did attempt exercises before surgery, but usually substituted simple exercise instructions for the more tangible biofeedback machine. Unfortunately, the success rate for incontinence correction without a biofeedback machine is only 50 percent.

In 1975, sexologist John D. Perry, Ph.D., one of the researchers and authors of *The G-Spot*, resurrected the work of Dr. Kegel. He spent twenty years developing the Perry Perineometer, a high-tech version of Kegel's biofeedback machine, which uses electromagnetic sensors and a computer to read out sophisticated measurements of the PC muscles' strength. Thousands of clinics around the country now use this device. His revival of Dr. Kegel's biofeedback program has spawned self-help clinics for the treatment of incontinence around the country. Attitudes have changed as well, and the U.S. Governmental Agency for Healthcare Research and Quality officially recommended in its 1992 report that doctors try biofeedback and other behavioral methods before resorting to drugs and surgery for incontinence. An at-home version of the perineometer is available from Dr. Perry's website (see Resources).

Strong and healthy PC muscles increase orgasmic response and aid female ejaculation, as well as help to cure urinary stress incontinence and a variety of other ills. Sexual taboos and stigmas and negative sexual events have created a reluctance in most women to become aware of and make use of their PC muscles, which causes the muscles to get out of shape or become chronically tense. Unfit PC muscles may be the culprit behind a wide range of reproductive health problems.

Female ejaculation has been misdiagnosed as urinary stress incontinence, surgical treatment for which includes cutting into the prostate gland. A hysterectomy may remove or damage the prostate. An episiotomy, the practice of cutting the vaginal opening to facilitate childbirth, cuts into the perineal sponge portion of the erectile tissue. The resulting scar tissue dampens sensitivity. Because the urethra was not considered part of the female sex organ and the female prostate was unrecognized, surgery in the past has been done without any knowledge that it could impair women's sexual response.

Dr. Zaviacic's studies indicated that female ejaculate may provide a soothing, protective agent for the urethra against "the ravages of urine," and possibly for the vagina as well. When one considers that 50 percent of visits by women to the gynecologist's office are for bladder and vaginal infections, and that 20 percent of these visits are for chronic infections (3 to 12 a year), it is clear that something is amiss in women's genitourinary system, and it is not because women are "not built right," as I have been told at the doctor's office. What is amiss is the condition of women's PC muscles. Tense PC muscles contribute to infections, because the lack of circulation creates a weakened vaginal and urethral environment that is an attractive home for infectious bacteria. Overly tense PC muscles can be caused by withholding one's ejaculate. Dr. Zaviacic's studies also noted the stagnation of ejaculate in the prostate in bed-ridden women with weak PC muscles.

In my video, *How to Female Ejaculate: Find Your G-Spot*, Dr. Bell talks about getting her PC muscles into shape:

> When I first started to learn how to ejaculate, I could barely squeeze my vaginal muscles. I started doing exercises, squeezing my pussy muscles together and then relaxing them. I did a hundred a session, three times a day. It took a few months, but after that I could shoot ejaculate across the room! My orgasms have improved, too!

Dr. Perry also created another electromagnetic device, the uterine myograph, which fits over the cervix and measures uterine muscle activity. He and Dr. Whipple identified a uterine muscle that works independently of the PC muscles. Interestingly, only a small minority of women could isolate the uterine muscles from the PC group. These important discoveries by Perry and Whipple were central to bringing a full picture of the muscles of the pelvic area into view.

☉ The G-Spot Nerve ☉

Because of the complexity of the human sex organs, and the muscles, nerves and brain that support them, orgasms and arousal can provide full-body sensations of intense erotic pleasure plus a wide range of emotions. The famous sexology studies of the past century underestimated the potential of the female orgasm, and therefore many individuals still don't fully understand or experience their orgasmic potential. Before *The G-Spot* authors Ladas, Whipple, and Perry researched female ejaculation and the G-spot, only the pudendal nerve, associated with the clitoris, the vulva, and the front one-third of the PC muscles, was considered to play a part in a woman's sexual response.

The pelvic nerve, by contrast, is connected to the urethra, the female prostate and g- spot, the bladder, uterus, and the back two-thirds of the PC muscles, including the uterine muscles. Both the pudendal and the pelvic nerves can stimulate an orgasm, but the orgasms are different. Although research is ongoing, the personal experiences of many women who clearly distinguish between a clitoral and G-spot orgasm suggest that the pelvic nerve may contribute to the more emotional experience of the G-spot orgasm.

Both the pudendal and the pelvic nerve are part of the 12th cranial nerve, the hypoglossal, which controls the motor nerve of the tongue. However, the vagus nerve, the 10th cranial nerve that controls sensory and motor functions, has also been implicated in G-spot orgasm. In 2002, Dr. Beverly Whipple, one of the researchers of *The G-Spot*, and B. R. Komisaruk published a paper in the *Journal of Sex and Marital Therapy*, Volume 28, entitled "Brain (PET) Responses to Vaginal-Cervical Self-Stimulation in Women with Complete Spinal Cord Injury." They used PET and MRI scans in order to identify that "the sensory vagus nerves are involved in input of sensations from the genitals to the brain, bypassing the spinal cord." They are now using fMRI to find out where in the brain orgasm takes place during vaginal-cervical stimulation. The vagus nerve also feeds the larynx, which, as we shall see in the next section, comes into play with the G-spot orgasm.

Both the 10th and 12th nerves, the hypoglossal and the vagus nerve, originate in the gray matter of the fourth ventricle of the medulla oblongata area of the brain stem. The medulla oblongata has remained virtually unchanged since the age of the Neanderthals; it controls sensory and motor skills, as well as our basic instincts for fleeing, fighting, feeding, and sexual pleasure. The cerebral cortex, in contrast, makes up the majority of the brain and controls fantasy, imagining, dreaming, and perhaps even consciousness. It is far less understood and well mapped than the medulla oblongata and other nerve centers of the "lower" brain or brain stem. However, it is well known that orgasms can take place without any sensory stimulation, as in dreams, and, for some individuals, through fantasy or the buildup of erotic energy alone. This indicates that orgasms, sexual pleasure, and erotic energy are also fueled by this more mysterious, and far less instinctual, part of the human brain.

Clearly we have more to learn about sexuality and this area of the brain. If the sexual, pelvic nerves connect to the area in the brain where scientists may one day find that consciousness resides, then one can barely fathom the potential for the untapped power source that is our sexual energy and pleasure.

⊚ Orgasms and Female Ejaculation ⊚

In the late 1800s, Freud expressed the view that the source of a mature woman's orgasmic response was the vagina. He argued that, in fact, clitoral orgasms belonged to adolescence and were therefore immature. This belief held sway for half a century, until sex researcher Alfred Kinsey turned the notion on its head. In his famous research in the early 1950s, he said that there is only one source of a woman's sexual response, and that is the clitoris. He argued that, in fact, the vagina has no nerve endings and is basically dead, empty space, and that its only function is to serve as a receptacle for the penis and sperm.

To this day, the supporters of Freud and Kinsey still argue about the true source of a woman's orgasm, with the vaginal proponents quite outshouted. But the notion of a unified female sex organ, put forward by Josephine Lowndes Sevely, renders obsolete these debates about which is the true female sexual center: the clitoris or the vagina. As it turns out, both these sexual centers are parts of one whole, functioning female sex organ.

Kinsey's conclusions created confusion for a significant group of sexologists, feminists, and individuals, women and men, about what, exactly, an orgasm is. Many women observed that their experiences did not match the "objective" observations and definitions of orgasm given by Kinsey and other researchers, especially Masters and Johnson.

Certainly, many feminists found Kinsey's work liberating. Women were no longer supposed to be dependent on intercourse to achieve orgasm. When the appalling news that a majority of women did not experience orgasm with their partners inspired feminists to brandish vibrators (and remove their bras) in the 1960s and 1970s, women set about exploring the uncharted territories of clitoral masturbation and orgasm. This led to the twentieth century's last explosion of sexual experimentation for women. Led by feminist sex educators such as Betty Dodson, author of *Sex for One*, and Del Williams and Joani Blank, founders of the first women-owned and -operated sexuality shops and mail-order companies, Eve's Garden and Good Vibrations, respectively, this movement achieved notable success in helping women claim their sexual autonomy. It also drastically lowered the number of women who could not achieve orgasm at all.

But some women simply didn't respond to clitoral stimulation, or were never able to achieve clitoral orgasm through intercourse. This problem, exacerbated by the Kinseysian emphasis on the clitoris, caused at least one doctor of sexology to throw up her hands and concede that perhaps women were never intended to have coital orgasms. Helen Kaplan describes just such a reaction in her book *The New Sex Therapy* (1974).

The women who took serious exception to Kinsey's definition of orgasm felt something was amiss. These women had experienced orgasms from penetration, but suddenly their orgasms were being called unattainable, impossible. For forty years their voices were drowned out by the orgiastic cries of joyful females reaching orgasm for the first time, thanks to their clitorises and a crew of battery-operated assistants. But some of them continued to speak. In her book *The Golden Notebook*, Doris Lessing asserted the existence of a vaginal orgasm and described its characteristics:

> A vaginal orgasm is emotion and nothing else, felt as emotion and expressed in sensations that are indistinguishable from emotion. The vaginal orgasm is a dissolving in a vague, dark generalized sensation like being swirled in a warm whirlpool.

In order to sort this matter out, sexologists Josephine and Irving Singer compiled a book, *The Goals of Human Sexuality* (1974), which collected and reported on many different experiences of female orgasm. They identified not one but three different types: clitoral, uterine, and blended.

The commonly recognized clitoral orgasm is also known as a vulvic orgasm. It is characterized by involuntary, rhythmic contractions of the PC muscles and does not require penetration. Multiple orgasms and insatiable feelings occur most easily with this type of orgasm.

The uterine orgasm is subjectively experienced as deeply emotional, involving no rhythmic contractions of the PC muscles. The measurable emotional changes that characterize the uterine orgasm involve emotional expression—making sounds—and the "apnea response." This apnea response causes the larynx to temporarily suspend the breath during orgasm and then to exhale it explosively, as occurs with other emotional reactions, such as laughing, sobbing, yawning, or screaming, providing the same release of tension. The uterine orgasm is dependent upon deep and rapid thrusts that jostle the cervix, which stimulates a large, sensitive membrane (called the peritoneum) which lines the abdomen and protects the organs of the abdomen and pelvic area, including the uterus. The uterine orgasm is most frequently a single, deeply satiating orgasm. This orgasm is rarely experienced by most women.

A blended orgasm combines elements of the clitoral and uterine orgasms. This is commonly called a "vaginal" or "G-spot" orgasm. A blended orgasm combines the involuntary contractions of the PC muscles that occur with the clitoral orgasm AND the feelings of deeper physical and emotional satisfaction that occur with the uterine orgasm. The apnea response at the moment of orgasm often occurs with the blended orgasm, although it is less pronounced than in the uterine orgasm. Multiple orgasms can occur in the blended orgasm, or one orgasm can feel like it is enough.

How the PC muscles operate during these three different types of orgasms to facilitate ejaculation is interesting. In the clitoral orgasm, the vagina balloons upward. In the blended orgasm, however, the vagina compresses downward and causes the PC muscles to push out the ejaculate. This pushing out, either from voluntary or involuntary action of the PC muscles, is what causes a woman to ejaculate. In the uterine orgasm, studies on how the muscles facilitate ejaculation, or don't, still need to be undertaken.

When *The G-Spot* authors Whipple and Perry used Perry's uterine myograph to study the PC muscles, their research provided physiological evidence for the Singers' report. They performed two tests—one to measure the pelvic muscle contractions with a clitoral orgasm (clitoral stimulation only), and one to measure the pelvic muscle contractions with a blended orgasm (simultaneous clitoral and G-spot stimulation).

The tests revealed that the PC muscles are active in a clitoral orgasm and the uterine muscles are nearly inactive. This indicates the pudendal nerve is activating the front third of the PC muscles during orgasm. In a blended orgasm, the PC muscles are much more active than in a clitoral orgasm. In addition, the uterine muscles become very active. This indicates a separate nerve, the pelvic nerve, is activating the back two-thirds of the PC muscles and the uterine muscle.

The results of the myograph gave physiological proof of Whipple and Perry's "two nerve" theory of female sexual response. Having two nerves that directly affect the female genitals means female orgasm can be triggered by either nerve, or by both simultaneously, with a whole spectrum of orgasmic responses between the two extremes.

THE DIFFERENT TYPES OF ORGASMS

	Clitoral	**Blended**	**Uterine**
Other names:	vulvic or vaginal	G-spot	none
Nerves:	pudendal	pudendal and pelvic	pelvic
Emotions:	mild	mild to intense	intense to "earth shattering"
Muscles:	first one-third of PC muscles	back two-thirds of PC muscles and uterine muscles	uterine muscles
Technique:	rapid stimulation of clitoris	stimulation of G-spot from slow to faster	deep thrusting that jostles the cervix
Ejaculation:	very difficult or impossible	easy	possible

Author and sexologist Dr. Carol Queen appeared in my video, *How to Female Ejaculate: Find Your G-Spot,* explaining what these three orgasms feel like to her, and how they affect her ability to ejaculate:

> I have had the experience of ejaculating with a vibrator on my clitoris, and I figured out what I must be doing is externally stimulating my 'urethral sponge' (G-spot). Sometimes this method results in ejaculation. However, ejaculation *always* occurs if I have something inside my vagina stimulating my G-spot, like my fingers, a dildo, or a penis. I think of the G-spot orgasm as a clitoral and vaginal orgasm all rolled into one; a blending of the two.
>
> But I have uterine orgasms that feel different from either of those. They are likely to happen when I'm connected deeply to someone and doing more Tantric-type methods that enhance my connection to my partner. Then my whole body gets involved and goes into waves of pleasure and my uterus will contract.

Dr. Queen believes that "the more one masturbates, the more different things one can find that will be true for them. That's why I call mine an orgasmic repertoire, because I know I have different types of orgasms."

⟲ All Women Have the Anatomy to Ejaculate ⟲

As we have learned in this chapter, the vast majority of women, like men, come out of the womb with a sex organ that equips them perfectly for both reproduction and sexual pleasure following sexual maturity. The female sex organ (defined in this book as the vulva, vagina, clitoris, urethra, prostate, pelvic muscles and nerves, and erectile tissue) has far more erectile tissue than was once thought, and it has a prostate that ejaculates fluid. It is similar in size and function to the male sex organ (defined in this book as the penis, testicles and scrotum, urethra, prostate, pelvic muscles and nerves, and erectile tissue), although its parts are arranged differently. The muscles that support the female sex organ need to be fit and healthy, and the nerves that enliven it are ready to do their job of providing more breadth and depth of sexual pleasure and emotional experience than once considered possible.

We have also learned the problems, some of them serious, that arise from a lack of information about the female prostate, and the real nature and extent of the woman's sex organ. For example, lack of muscle fitness has caused far too many gynecological problems for women.

We have seen how, since it is not commonly known that women have a prostate, this locus of sexual pleasure has been overlooked. The vagina has been considered unfeeling, the clitoris has been overvalued, and the urethra seen as something that divides the clitoris and vagina into two parts, rather than the centerpiece (because it houses the G-spot) of the whole female sex organ.

Many scientific and personal discoveries during the past twenty years have contributed to uncovering the workings of female ejaculation. All of these, at every step, flew in the face of longheld cultural views and behavior. In the next chapter, we'll learn how other cultures have accepted and celebrated female ejaculation, and come to a greater appreciation of our own feminine waters.

CHAPTER THREE

The Ancient Herstory of Female Ejaculation

NATALIE'S FANTASY: Natalie had recently broken up with her beloved of seven years, and her pain was unbearable. She dearly missed the closeness and the deep, satisfying lovemaking they shared. She had been on the verge of opening her sense of touch and her heart to new levels when he'd left. To even think of lovemaking now sent a searing pain up her arms, like the skin was being stripped from her bones. She needed serious comfort. She had heard of ancient temples in India, where erotic love at its highest level had been worshipped, and she let herself imagine the healing power that such a place could hold for her....

Upon stepping onto the sacred grounds one moonlit evening, she looked around, then headed toward a little nook where a voluptuous female figure with a large vulva was carved in the rock. Natalie fell down on her knees, begging a higher power for comfort and praying for guidance. As if in answer, she was overcome with erotic pleasure and a warm, melting love that left her feeling open and soft. She meditated on this sensation, while she sat cross-legged, breathing deeply and squeezing her pelvic muscles. Her swollen vulva grew warm and then hot. She felt flushed with ejaculate.

She removed a large seashell from her bag and squatted over it. She intended to collect her ejaculate, for the first time, in order to experience its rejuvenating qualities. As she massaged her vulva and "sacred spot" while staying focused on the open and loving feeling, her ejaculate streamed out into the shell bowl. She poured the waters over her

upturned, moonlit face, praying to the Goddess of Love and Healing to keep her sensuality strong and open to change, as she mourned the loss of the man she once loved.

As the sweet nectar ran down her face and glistened on her naked breasts, her heart felt free and full of peace. She left the temple site noticing her constant emotional pain was absent, replaced by an excitement for what her future might hold for her.

Knowledge of female ejaculation is by no means new. Cultures around the world have left records showing that they knew of its existence, and viewed it as natural, normal, and, in some cases, healing and sacred. The openness of some of these cultures toward female ejaculation illustrates how modern Western society is actually unusual in its ignorance about these feminine "flowing waters."

Knowing more about how female ejaculation was looked upon by other societies can help to dispel the view of female ejaculation as an abnormality, and offer insight into its erotic, healing, and sacred aspects. From this, a new attitude can be developed, one that is helpful to individuals and couples today and encourages social acceptance of this phenomenon.

In addition to considering older, more metaphysical views about the role female ejaculation plays in reproduction and how it may be used for rejuvenation and healing, this chapter will also discuss how some modern-day practitioners are putting these old beliefs back in practice.

Translations of the ancient texts in which information on female ejaculation can be found were often distorted, and sections were deleted by translators for whom the concepts were unfamiliar or contrary to their belief systems. Some sources may have used the terms "urine" or "emissions" where the term "female ejaculation" is more accurate. If, in the future, academic researchers go back over the texts looking for information regarding female ejaculation, more information is certain to be revealed.

For now, the pieces that have surfaced are telling. I have collected these fragments in one place in the hope that the colorful herstory of female ejaculation will encourage our own culture to borrow from and build upon this information—as Natalie was inspired to do in the imaginative story above. Creating our own erotic contexts, healing uses, and sacred expressions to honor female ejaculation will help us understand and relate to these ancient beliefs about the feminine waters.

☺ *Liquor Vitae*—Ancient Greece and Rome ☺

From 600 B.C. to A.D. 200, the origin of female ejaculation in the body and its role in reproduction were explored by many classical philosophers and physicians from Pythagoras to Hippocrates, from Aristotle to Galen. What was not debated was its existence. In fact, female ejaculation was a fact of life for the Greeks and Romans. They named the inner labial lips, from which these fluids flowed, the *nymphea,* or "water goddesses." Galen gives a lusty and useful view of female ejaculation in his treatise *On the Usefulness of the Parts of the Body:*

> This liquid not only stimulates the sexual act but also is able to give pleasure and moisten the passageway as it escapes. It manifestly flows from women as they experience the greatest pleasure in coitus, when it is perceptibly shed upon the male pudendum; indeed, such an outflow seems to give a certain pleasure even to eunuchs.

The Greeks and Romans believed that both male and female fluids were seminal and that men and women equally contributed their "seeds" to the creation of life. These fluids, called by the Romans *liquor vitae,* contained vital essences that were considered not only rejuvenating to the body but essential to the creation of life.

Hippocrates believed that the female essence must mix with the male essence in order for new, human life to be created. This belief in its reproductive importance was rejected by Aristotle, who nevertheless recognized its existence. He claimed, however, that the male essence alone was responsible for conception, and that the female essence was responsible solely for the physical nourishment of the fetus.

These two views vied for prominence for 500 years, until Galen, a Greek-born physician known as the "father of medicine," proposed a new formula. He supported his predecessors' views that both male and female essences were needed to contribute to conception, to the creation of new life, though not, as Aristotle believed, to gestation. Galen argued that, after playing its role in conception, the female fluid could not nourish the fetus in the womb because it was too "cold." As in Chinese medicine, the Greeks and Romans used the concepts of hot and cold to convey certain functional characteristics of the body and of gender. Galen again describes female ejaculate:

> Since the female is more frigid than the male, the fluid in her prostate is unconcocted and thin. This contributes nothing to the generation [gestation] of offspring.

•

Following her extensive, Harvard University–funded research on the history of female ejaculation in the West, Josephine Lowndes Sevely reported on these beliefs and other findings about female ejaculation in her book, *Eve's Secrets*. What her work, and a consideration of classical texts, tells us is that female ejaculation was not only recognized by the classical philosophers and scientists, but also that they debated and discussed its properties in detail.

◌ *Nectar of the Gods*—Ancient India ◌

We know that *amrita*, the "nectar of the gods," was honored as a sacred female erotic fluid in some parts of India. About a thousand years ago, a spiritual tradition known as Tantra flourished in central and eastern India, and it considered sexuality as a powerful tool for spiritual enlightenment. The sexual act was seen as an art and a sacred ritual, and there were more than eighty-five temples devoted to the worship of divine sexual energy.

The Tantric temples were decorated with life-size statues of individuals, couples, and groups in highly complex and physically difficult erotic positions—positions that the study of certain forms of hatha yoga, which are an integral part of Tantra, makes attainable over time. A typical Western perception of such temples, and perhaps the only feasible Western interpretation of such behavior, is of a free-for-all bacchanal. However, this is a gross misconception.

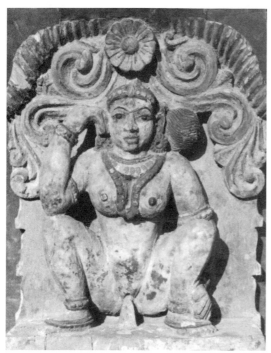

A statue depicting female "emissions" from an ancient Tantric temple at Karnataka, India.

Courtesy Nik Douglas. Reprinted from his book, *Spiritual Sex*

Practitioners of Tantra believed that sexual energy is an embodiment of divine energy, and that this energy can be intensified and carried through the body by the breath, setting every nerve on erotic fire. They developed hours-long rituals of enhanced techniques and positions to heighten the senses to their fullest. Their goal was to use sex as a vehicle for enlightenment and attain an altered state of cosmic unity through extended orgasms.

Since sex was viewed and used as a highly spiritual expression, it is no surprise that one of its physical manifestations, ejaculate fluid, would also be viewed as spiritual and studied in detail. In his book *Spiritual Sex* Nik Douglas explains that Siddha Yoga teachings on Tantric sex discuss three distinct types of female emission: the *suratham* (winelike juice), the *sronithram* (blood-tinged emission), and the *suklam* (ejaculate). It also makes sense that arousing a woman properly and satisfying her sexually was integral to the sacred erotic practice, to ensure that these emissions are secreted. The teachings explain that by doing so, the three fluids are secreted in sequence. Douglas tells us:

> The "lotus nectar" of the precious consort, released by her as an embodiment of the Great Goddess during a high rite of Tantric sex, can have a wide variety of flavors, each credited with specific transcendental and magical properties.

Tantric teaching encourages people to drink these emissions, a practice called *amaroli*, because they are full of healthy ingredients, such as hormones, vitamins, and minerals. Douglas continues:

> Many Tantras recommend amaroli as a high sacrament, stating that the [emissions] be drunk directly "from the lips of the Yoni" (vulva) at the culmination of intimacy.

The "Tantras" referred to are writings by yogic sages that predate the tenth century Tantric temples by a thousand years. Some of these teachings had detailed descriptions of the characteristics and use of female ejaculation.

The Hindu culture also gave us a remarkable text on the art of love-making, *The Kama Sutra*, written over two thousand years ago. *The Kama Sutra* is well known to Westerners because it was "discovered" and translated by the famous Victorian explorer, poet, and scholar, Sir Richard Burton. Chapters of it are devoted to the practical aspects of lovemaking. In the original text written by the yogic sage Vatsyayana, female ejaculation is mentioned in a context that seems to echo the view of the ancient Greeks—that female ejaculate contains seed: "The semen of women continues to fall from the beginning of the sexual union to its end, in the same way as that of the male."

From these Indian traditions and texts, we see that female ejaculation was well known, acknowledged for the health-giving properties of its contents, and used in sacred religious practices that utilized sexual energy. Another interesting use for female ejaculate occurred in ancient China, as we shall soon see.

⑥ *The Third Water*—The Taoist Tradition ◉

The 2,500-year-old Chinese scientific and philosophical tradition of Taoism views female ejaculation as sacred and essential to life. Like Tantra in ancient India, Taoism has a "three water" view of female ejaculation, and it also links the three types of female emission to corresponding levels of stimulation and arousal in women. Master Mantak Chia, a Buddhist monk who teaches and resides in the Chiang Mai province of Thailand, is renowned for bringing the ancient Taoist secrets of lovemaking to the West via his book *Taoist Secrets of Love: Cultivating Male Sexual Energy.* He has the following to say regarding the discussion of female ejaculation in the ancient Taoist texts:

> The ancient Taoists regarded the woman's fluids as being vital both for herself and her man. The First Water is the lubricant that begins the feeling of Arousal; it "deepens the water and widens the river." This fulfills a "golden rule" of Taoist sexual respect: "Never launch the boat on a rocky river!"

> The rule refers to respecting the time of Yin, the time of Water, the time that is necessary for the Jade Cavern's preparations to receive. We can think of this Water like the man's "Happy Drops"; this clear lubricant is often seen early in lovemaking with the erection and serves to blend with the woman's First Water and further lubricate the vagina.

> The Second Water is the Water of Higher Arousal, the beginning of orgasm. The woman is fully engaged in a climbing sensual and sexual excitement. "The river flows."

> The Third Water comes with the height of orgasm; it's what we think of as the female ejaculation and completes the internal balance of Water and Fire (*Kan* and *Li*) in the woman and in the couple. "The river overflows its banks flooding the fields with life-giving nourishment!"

Marina is a midwife who works in many countries, including Russia, Thailand and Israel. A waterbirth and baby yoga pioneer, she encourages the mixing of the male and female essences and the Third Water during the birth process. She says:

> Not only does this lubricate the passageway and relax the pelvic muscles to ease the birthing process, but the baby is delivered into the world by the ejaculatory waters.

Exactly how the "essence" that is in female ejaculate (the essence that the ancients believed played a role in reproduction) is transmitted other than through energy pathways may have a modern, scientific explanation. As we learned in Chapter 2 in the section "What *Is* Female Ejaculate?," scientists have discovered that tiny amounts of ejaculate continually seep from the female prostate into the vagina, creating a nurturing environment for sperm—a reversal of the prevailing view of the vagina as a hostile environment for sperm.

☺ *Ejaculation Bowls*—16th Century Japan ☺

Female ejaculation pours, streams, falls, and overflows in some ancient traditions, and sixteenth century Japan elevated the event to an art form. For two centuries the *shunga* artistic movement flourished there, celebrating sensual pleasures and sexual delights in explicit, prolific detail on woodblock prints. The prints depicted implements to increase and collect the sought-after female fluids with an imagination and a graphic detail that would surely make a Victorian faint, and even our modern, sexually open society blush.

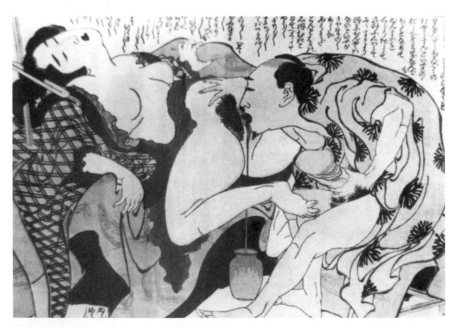

A Japanese Woodcut Depicting a Man Holding a Container to Catch Female Ejaculate
reprinted from *Erotique du Japon*

Yet the woodcuts from this period give undeniable proof that, for Japanese society in this period, female ejaculation not only existed, it was desired, celebrated, and enjoyed in every detail. In keeping with celebrating the pure physical enjoyment of sensual pleasures, the Japanese considered female ejaculation an aphrodisiac. They believed it had rejuvenating qualities as well, and encouraged that it be drunk, for its supposed ability to reverse the aging process.

In his book, the title of which translates as *The Third Dimension of Lust: The Secrets of Female Ejaculation*, Austrian professor of sexology Dr. Karl Stifter tells us that a Japanese woman who wanted to generate the ejaculate fluid by herself used a special instrument called the *heikonoinho,* or dildo. She would masturbate until she had an orgasm, and would catch the ejaculate in a container. Another ejaculate vessel, called a *harikata,* was a bowl with a dildo and incense holder attached to it. She could stimulate herself with the dildo and then catch her ejaculate fluid in the basin.

Dr. Stifter also describes another instrument used by Japanese women for self-pleasuring, which could be tied to the woman's foot so she could easily satisfy herself. Usually made of buffalo or oxen horn, the instrument was hollow inside and could be warmed before use. Scraps of silk were stuffed into the hollow horn to catch and absorb the feminine waters. Later, hot water was poured over the silk contents. After steeping, the water was drunk as tea for its healthful properties.

⊚ *Amplexus Reservaturs*—The Catholic Tradition ⊚ in Medieval Europe

While not often considered a tradition that embraced sensuality, it is known that priests of the Catholic Church were instructed for centuries to counsel couples to avoid *amplexus reservaturs,* practices believed to lead to the suppression of semination by *both* sexes (the same was true for *coitus interruptus,* diversion of male semen from the womb). This ban had its roots in medieval times, but continues in the Catholic Church to this day, as this notice, entitled "Acta Apostolicae Sedis," demonstrates. The notice, dated 30 June 1952, was issued by the Holy Office, and is translated in the Irish Ecclesiastical Record:

> In their work of the care of souls and the direction of consciences
> [priests] should never, either spontaneously or in reply to a question,
> presume so to speak of the *amplexus reservatus* as if there were no
> objection to it from the standpoint of Christian law.

Obviously, the Greek idea of a female seed being part of conception and procreation survived into medieval times, whereupon it was declared a sin by the Roman Catholic Church for a woman to *not* ejaculate!

⟲ *The Waters of Gaia*—Indigenous Peoples ⟲

Harley Thunder Strikes SwiftDeer Reagan is a Metis Cherokee Native American, of the Twisted Hair shaman tradition. He was the last one of his lineage, during the early 1950s, to receive the initiation into the mysteries he calls *Quodoushka*, "sacred sexual union." A Twisted Hair shaman is one who follows his own traditions but also incorporates many others. In modern times, performing his calling as a Twisted Hair means studying other cultures around the world, something not possible two hundred years ago for a Native American.

SwiftDeer's travels have taken him to India, South Africa, and around Asia and Europe to speak with the shamans of surviving native cultures or to study the ruins and texts of native cultures destroyed long ago. In his book, *Song of the Deer: The Great Sundance Journey of the Soul*, he discusses these Quodoushka teachings and his years of travel.

Quodoushka teaches that female ejaculation "represents a woman's ability to be (comfortable) in her masculine side," and that it represents a "free, individual, and autonomous woman totally owning her orgasmic power and potential." SwiftDeer spoke to me about female ejaculation in a telephone conversation:

> Although three of the six genital anatomy types that Quodoushka
> distinguishes between have a dispositional nature to ejaculate, any
> woman can learn how. What is needed most is presence of mind

toward the task and an awareness about a woman's ability to ejaculate. The biggest stumbling blocks to learning are being embarrassed by urine and the subconscious suppression of it, which shuts female ejaculation down. People are skittish around bodily fluids due to AIDS and attitudes, but in a committed, loving, monogamous relationship, there is no need to fear.

When I asked him if his culture had the "Three Waters" view of female erotic fluids and the idea of essences, to my surprise he said yes on both counts:

The three waters are vaginal secretions and the "Dew Drops" from the mouth of the cervix, which when mixed are called the "Mist of the Red Lion" or "*Jacquer*." When the Mist is added to the ejaculate fluid, called the "Flood of Venus," what you have is the "Elixir of Life." This elixir is a measurement of one's *orende* or *chi*.

The African shamans of the Dagara and the Zulu of South Africa told SwiftDeer that the Three Waters is an important part of their concepts as well. SwiftDeer also confirmed that Quodoushka believes female ejaculate contains hormones and minerals, and "that it is healthful and life affirming."

While reading what is currently known about historical attitudes toward female ejaculation for this book, I was disappointed that nothing seemed to have been discovered or documented in the Celtic tradition, so I decided to do a little research of my own. My first suspect was the goddess Shiela-na-Gig, due to the typical depiction of her holding open her greatly exaggerated vulva. I looked through many pictures of her stone images for signs of flowing waters, but in the end found nothing, save an exceptionally researched thesis about Sila na Geige (a.k.a. Shiela-na-Gig) by researcher and writer Kathryn Price.

When I contacted Price regarding the possibility of the Shiela-na-Gig ejaculating, she referred me to the myth of the Celtic goddess Morrigan. In her e-mail to me, she relayed what she recalled of this goddess:

The Morrigan is said to have created the River on Samhain after having sex with the Dagda (Earth God). The versions I've read said She

created it by urinating. But it would be interesting to go back to the
primary translations of that myth and see. Of course, one of the
problems we struggle with in researching the Celtic goddesses is
that there's a big misogyny filter. Usually the tales were written down
by early Christian monks, and sometimes their biases are really
obvious. The best research is when we can find a number of different
records of a tale—sometimes what one author/transcriber left
out, another one recorded.

When I mentioned this tale about the Celtic goddess Morrigan urinating
and creating the rivers to Harley SwiftDeer, he immediately cut in on my
recital of the tale and said:

> It's not "urinate!" She releases Gaia and creates the waters of life! She
> releases the "Everlasting Stream of Livingness." Water was life to the
> Celtic culture. Without water, we have no life.

> You see, ancient peoples, especially Celtic, spoke of these matters in
> the poetic, mythological legends and songs of their creation stories.
> They did not speak so practically about male and female ejaculate and
> taking it into one's mouth, for example.

> Celtic wisdom is buried in "sex magick" (sacred sex), which was also
> [replaced] by Christianity. The same is true for most Native Americans,
> who are now mostly Catholic and unaware of their tradition. Bodily
> secretions are equated with water, with life. In sex magick, we have the
> dark and light. The dark uses blood, related to death. The light uses
> the fluids that create life: male and female ejaculate.

SwiftDeer recounted a Quodoushka ceremony in which the female
bestows immortality upon the male by using her ejaculate. This occurs in
sacred sex when female ejaculate is combined with male fluid, specifically,
when he "takes her back," meaning she sits on his face and she ejaculates.
He puts his hands in a triangle over her womb and she puts hers in a triangle over his soft spot on top of his head. The essence is transferred to him
via energy and via the force of her ejaculate into his mouth. He drinks his
own ejaculate and hers:

> That is how a male receives immortality—through this "Kiss of Life."
> When ejaculate is shooting from the female, it is symbolic of her life
> force flowing out into the world, and that is related to the creation of
> the universe [in Quodoushka mythology].

When the Romans destroyed the ancient Western European tribal tradition, the divine feminine was lost. The powers of birth and spiritual rejuvenation promised by the feminine power, symbolized by the vulva, were no longer celebrated. The feminine healing power of ejaculate in sacred sex has likely been celebrated for many millennia. Temple priestesses in several ancient traditions, including the devadasi of India, and the priestesses of Isis in Egypt and of Innana in Sumeria, wed themselves to the service of healing men through the use of sacred sexual energy, which may have included female ejaculate.

Kenneth Ray Stubbs, Ph.D., editor of the anthology *Women of the Light,* offers a modern view of the lives of women who work in this capacity. In the book, nine contemporary women speak in their own voices about the rewards of their work, and their various approaches. Corynna Clarke is one such modern-day priestess of the healing, feminine aspect of sacred sexual energy. While being interviewed for my video *Tantric Journey to Female Orgasm: Awaken Your G-Spot,* she had this to say about her chosen vocation:

> My work is about healing the wounds inflicted by a violent society.
> Temple priestesses in ancient times viewed the ejaculate as a symbol
> of the goddess, and men came to the temple for healing their heads
> that were still at war. The priestess would wash them in the waters of
> the temple pool and the waters of the *amrita,* and help men move their
> energy from the warrior to the shaman by helping them deal with the
> pains of war, like dealing with post-traumatic stress syndrome. It is like
> a calling for me to do this kind of work. It never ceases to move my
> heart and soul when I hear the stories and see the process of recovery
> start to unfold.

When anthropologists, such as American Margaret Mead and German Otto Finsch, began to study indigenous cultures during the twentieth century, some indigenous tribespeople relayed their knowledge and practice of female ejaculation to Western researchers. Sevely and the authors of *The G-Spot* report that the Native-American Mohave, the Trukese of the Coral Islands of the South Pacific, and the Ponapese of the South Pacific, who called ejaculation "spraying the wall," are just a few of the surviving tribal cultures around the world where female ejaculation is viewed as a normal female body function. They may consider female ejaculate as having a role in reproduction, too. Otto Finsch tells us in his study of the Ponapese that "to impregnate his wife, a man must first stimulate her to the point where she 'urinates,' and only then proceed to have intercourse with her."

Though historical information on female ejaculation has been neglected, it has not been lost altogether. The roots of female ejaculation can be traced from antiquity to the present day. Surviving historical texts and oral traditions, as well as modern research, link us to ancient, cross-cultural recognition and acceptance of female ejaculation. The resurrection of this information has brought female ejaculation back into the modern-day bedroom and into Western consciousness in a celebratory and life-affirming way, closing a circle that has been broken too long. Together, the recent findings by Western researchers and the ancients' views on female ejaculation open up a whole new world of understanding in which to explore female ejaculation.

The next part of the book explains in hands-on detail how to bring female ejaculation into the bedroom, to explore and play with! Let's begin by getting down to the business of getting this incredibly luscious female spring working again.

techniques *for a*
FEMININE FOUNTAIN

CHAPTER FOUR

Ejaculate Without an Orgasm

Laura returned from a female ejaculation class sweaty and excited. She flopped down on the bed and pulled the clear plastic speculum from her purse. Images of the many G-spots she had seen kept flashing before her eyes. But the image that lingered the longest was that of her own G-spot. It was as if she couldn't believe that she possessed such a thing. She settled down on the floor, her back against the bed, her full-length mirror in front of her. She decided to have another look.

She inserted the speculum and turned it sideways. There it was. Her jaw dropped in amazement as her G-spot revealed itself again. She studied it for a while, then she touched it. She identified all the parts of her newly revealed sex organ: vagina, clitoris, G-spot, urethra, and vulva. She spent some time trying to imagine them as one organ. That was a little hard to do, so she removed the speculum and moved on to see if she remembered how to stimulate her G-spot.

She aroused herself and watched her vulva puff up, and noticed how her G-spot moved when she pushed with her PC muscles. She looked at her urethra buried in the folds, and began to understand how it was tied erotically to her vagina. She inserted her sex toy and was surprised at how much movement her urethra actually experienced during penetration. She shook her head. It was interesting to see it all this closely and to notice how all the parts worked together.

"Especially this ejaculation business," she thought, as she relaxed into the warm sensations of her G-spot, eager to see if she could get her ejaculate to flow.

Learning how to ejaculate is fairly easy. For those who want to learn, I've designed a practical approach that will increase your chances of achieving success—and you don't need to have an orgasm to do it! All you need is some privacy, a mirror, your finger, and the desire to learn.

I have heard from hundreds of women friends, acquaintances, and those who have attended my G-spot workshops or lectures on female ejaculation. I have spoken to women at conferences, through correspondence about my videos, and in passing conversations. My most memorable "in-transit" conversation took place with a stranger at a rest stop in a remote mountain pass, before each of us headed out again on our solitary travels. After hearing so many women's remarks and stories over the years, I have observed that positive attitudes correlate to a woman's success in learning to ejaculate. Therefore, this chapter begins by checking your mental and physical readiness for ejaculation.

This check-in is followed by step-by-step instructions for finding your G-spot and stimulating it to make your juices flow. Then you will learn a basic technique for ejaculating without an orgasm, which will give you a solid base for understanding the mechanics involved in ejaculating, as well as the thrill of actually experiencing it! These solo explorations will prepare you for integrating female ejaculation successfully into orgasms (Chapter 5) and into sexual relations with a partner (Chapter 6).

Let's begin by "checking under the hood" and understanding how the three Ms—mental attitude, muscle strength, and menstrual cycle—affect your ability to learn how to ejaculate. Good luck!

☉ The Right Mental Attitude ☉

Attitude is important in learning how to ejaculate. It is essential that you feel ready. I have identified six general attitudes women hold toward female ejaculation. You may fall into one category or another, or you may overlap between a few categories. Wherever you fit, remember that your thoughts and feelings are perfectly normal. However you feel right now about female ejaculation, if you really want to learn to ejaculate, you will.

ဢ A handful of women seem to simply need to hear the words "female ejaculation" and they will ejaculate the next day, as if all they needed was permission. These women illustrate how easy female ejaculation can be, once we believe we can do it.

ဢ Some other women remember a time from their early years when they ejaculated, thought it odd, never did it again, and forgot about it. In their first attempts at being sexual, their bodies did something they just blocked out. The glazed look that comes across their faces as they remember tells me they have been transported back in time and are wondering who that early sexual being was and what has happened to her. These women illustrate how we have learned to modify our sexual behavior by controlling and withholding ejaculation.

Other gals are eager to ejaculate, and try and try, but have no success. This group gets an "A" for effort and enthusiasm in my book. Their struggles are genuine and earnest, and I urge them to continue. Generally, this group falls into one of the following two categories:

ဢ Some of these women are inexperienced with communication and sexual technique, and may suffer from leftover adolescent embarrassment or culturally induced shame about looking at and talking about their bodies. They, and their partners, don't know quite how to navigate the body and touch it for maximum erotic effect, or have not yet learned to communicate this knowledge to one another. They illustrate how discomfort with our bodies and lack of skill with touch and communicating about touch can inhibit ejaculation.

Other women eager to ejaculate have difficulty doing so because of serious psychological issues about the body and sexuality. These problems can require a fair amount of complicated inner work. For example, deep-seated tension in the body can result from carrying around unresolved emotional or psychological issues, and this tension can block the relaxation that facilitates ejaculation. They illustrate how unresolved sexual issues or discomfort with their present sexual situation can inhibit ejaculation.

Then there are the ladies who already ejaculate. They are excited to share their experiences and pick up some tips. They appear proud and happy with their accomplishments. They illustrate the freedom and sense of confidence that often emerge when we claim our ejaculatory birthright.

The last category of women, frequent callers when I appear on radio shows, are upset by the news that women can and do ejaculate. Agitated because they feel pressured to ejaculate, they vehemently question the existence of female ejaculation. I interpret this rejection as denial. I sympathize with their shock and surprise, but I emphatically declare the reality of women's ability to ejaculate. These women illustrate how denial, ignorance, and resistance can thwart attempts to ejaculate.

The first step in learning to ejaculate is identifying your mental attitude toward ejaculation—your "ejaculation readiness." Your heart is the best indicator of whether you are ready. If you are unsure, take this quick test to see where you stand. Rate each question on a 1–5 scale, scoring 5 for a strong yes and 1 for an emphatic no.

CHECKING UNDER THE HOOD: AN ATTITUDE TEST

I. I like the idea of female ejaculation.

2. I understand that "holding back" controls my ability to ejaculate.

3. I am comfortable with my body and with touching it.

4. I am comfortable expressing emotions during sex.

5. I believe female ejaculation is accessible to me.

6. I feel that I could "let go and let it flow."

7. I want the freedom and confidence that comes with owning my ability to ejaculate.

SCORE:
35–27: Green light.   **26–14:** Proceed with caution.   **13–7:** Stop and wait.

If you scored a "green light," your attitude is open and confident, and you will probably ejaculate without much effort. If you scored "proceed with caution," your attitude is lukewarm and your chances are fifty-fifty, but you'll learn much in your attempts to ejaculate. If you scored "stop and wait," you probably have reservations that will create problems ejaculating, and it is best to realize that you may not be ready yet to take this on. If you do, you might just frustrate yourself and create more obstacles to overcome next time.

If you scored a "green light" or "proceed with caution," take the physical readiness tests which follow. If you scored "stop and wait," continue to read the rest of the book: Chapter 8 in particular may be of help to you. Those lukewarm about or resistant to the idea of ejaculation may find that the best approach is to finish the book, wait awhile and let the information simmer, then retake the test. Remember, learning to ejaculate is your choice and yours alone.

⊙ PC Muscle Strength and Flexibility ⊙

Next, let's determine if you are physically ready to learn to ejaculate, by testing the strength of your pelvic muscles. Toned pubococcygeus (PC) muscles play an important role in a woman's ability to ejaculate. These pelvic muscles need to be strong and toned to allow sexual energy to flow freely, but they are often tense or weak. When I taught How to Strip for Your Lover classes, I saw too many women having difficulty doing a simple bump and grind. The reason for this is often embarrassment about moving in an erotic way: This same embarrassment can contribute to allowing the PC muscles to become weak or tense.

Weak PC muscles get out of shape from lack of use, and like any muscles that are underused, they shrink. Atrophied pelvic muscles can cause a variety of problems, such as displaced internal organs, difficulty in childbirth, urinary stress incontinence, and even inability to achieve orgasm. The force, and possibly the quantity, of ejaculation is reduced in women who have weak PC muscles.

Tense PC muscles can be triggered by negative sexual encounters, and the condition can be chronic. Tense muscles can cause painful menstrual cramps, vaginal dryness, and vaginal and urinary tract infections, and can even be mistaken for lower-back pain. Because women tighten this muscle to shut off the flow of ejaculate and stop the sensations that precede ejaculation, tense muscles are just as common in women who don't ejaculate as are weak muscles. Tense PC muscles can also prevent or impair orgasm.

Both conditions affect circulation in the genital area. Tense muscles can cut off circulation, much like white knuckles on a tight fist. Flabby muscles also diminish circulation. A chronically constricted blood supply causes problems that can progress to disease over time. Fifty percent of visits to the gynecologist's office are for bladder and vaginal infections. Twenty percent of those women have chronic infections, often suffering from three to a dozen infections a year. I believe unfit PC muscles contribute to this high rate of infection.

Simple awareness and exercise can correct lack of PC-muscle fitness and prevent serious health problems. As we all know, body awareness and exercise have incredible benefits, and even if you already use exercise and diet to maintain your health, you should consider adding a PC-muscle strengthening regimen to your routines. Fit PC muscles will help your G-spot become an elaborate web of electrifying sensations and pulsating pleasures that keep the waters flowing.

CHECKING UNDER THE HOOD: MUSCLE STRENGTH AND FLEXIBILITY TESTS

The best way to test the strength and flexibility of your PC muscles is to use a biofeedback instrument at home, such as the perineometer, and/or visit a clinic that uses this instrument. Some health clinics also offer the assistance of trained professionals who can select the best exercises for you and guide you in using them. (See the section "The PC Muscles" in Chapter 2 for more on how perineometers work, and consult the Resources section in the back of the book for health clinics that may use them.) Your urologist may be able to recommend a clinic. However, since these clinics are still scarce, I've developed a test for use at home.

PC Muscles Flexibility Test

First, test the flexibility of your PC muscles by inserting *your finger up to the first joint* (use lube if you'd like) inside the opening of your vagina. Squeeze your finger with your PC muscles and determine which of the following is the most appropriate description of your sensation:

1. The vaginal opening is very relaxed and open when I first insert my finger, and I cannot squeeze my finger. (Score 1)

2. The vaginal opening is very relaxed and open when I first insert my finger. I can squeeze my finger, but it still does not appear to be snug. (Score 2)

3. The vaginal opening snugly encases my finger but does not feel tight. I can squeeze my finger with my PC muscles. (Score 3)

~ *How to Measure the Strength and* ~ *Flexibility of Your PC Muscles*

You can test both the strength and flexibility of your PC muscles using your sense of touch, with finger joints and finger widths as measures. I recommend doing this test more than once. The results of your first test may be confusing, and your score may change as you become more acquainted with the tests and with the PC muscles. Therefore, use your score as a general guide, and not a strict rule.

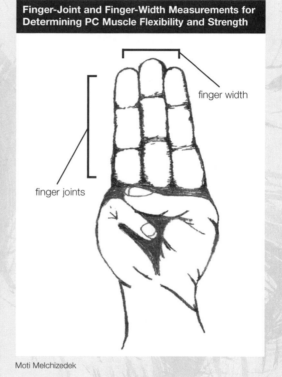

Finger-Joint and Finger-Width Measurements for Determining PC Muscle Flexibility and Strength

finger width

finger joints

Moti Melchizedek

4. The vaginal opening feels very tight, but allows entrance of my finger. I can push on my vagina, toward my anus, and feel the vaginal opening loosen. (Score 4)

5. The vaginal opening is too tight to insert my finger. (Score 5)

FLEXIBILITY SCORE:

1–2: Weak.   **3:** Normal.   **4–5:** Tense.

PC Muscles Strength Test

Next, test the strength of your PC muscles. To do this, you must find them. They are a band of muscles that lies deep inside the vagina. Lie back, resting on one elbow, and bend the opposite knee. Place your feet wherever they feel most comfortable. Moisten your forefinger (use lube if it feels better) and insert it into your vagina up to the *third finger joint*. Locate a band of muscles by feeling the muscle band on the right- and left-side walls of the vagina, as well as along the bottom (toward the anus). Here's a tip: Imagine a clock face, with the roof of the vagina at twelve and floor of the vagina at six. In general, at two and ten o'clock, the pelvic bone is quite noticeable when your finger is two joints in. The muscles lie just beyond the bone at a three finger-joint depth. Squeeze and relax your muscles to help identify them.

Once you have found and explored this band of muscles, you are ready to measure its width using the width of your fingers (see sidebar and illustration on the previous page for help). Explore these muscles further and get acquainted with them, as you would with muscles elsewhere in your body, by massaging, pushing, and probing. Contract these muscles and feel with your finger how they bulge and move. See whether they are wider when you relax them and narrower when you contract them. Now, measure the width of the band of muscles. Is it as thin as a pencil, or as thick as three fingers, or somewhere in between? Score your answer below:

Strength Score: One finger width: weak (Score 1).
Three finger widths: normal (Score 3).
Two finger widths: tense (Score 5).

Add the Muscle Flexibility Test score and the Muscle Strength Test score together.

Overall Score: 2–3: Weak.   6: Normal.   9–10: Tense.

If you scored "normal," your muscles are in good shape for ejaculation. If you scored "tense," your muscles may be strong enough to aid ejaculation, but they may have become tense because you've been unconsciously stopping your ejaculate flow. You may experience some difficulty ejaculating until you recondition your muscles to relax more fully. If you scored "weak," you may find it difficult to ejaculate until you build up more strength in your PC muscles. You'll learn how to do this below. Whatever your score is, you will benefit from reading and practicing the exercises for PC muscles that follow.

If you scored "weak" or "tense," read and practice the exercises below, and continue on with the next section about finding your G-spot. You may still be able to ejaculate now, simply by being aware of the state of your PC muscles. If you experience problems with the ejaculatory exploration exercises, work with the PC muscle exercises below for a few weeks and then try ejaculating again.

EXERCISES TO BUILD HEALTHY PC MUSCLES

These exercises will help weak muscles become stronger, tense muscles become relaxed, and healthy muscles maintain their strength and flexibility. Feeling the difference may take one to six weeks, but don't despair. PC muscles shape up quickly and improvements are soon noticeable.

Exercise for Weak PC Muscles

Choose something to squeeze against, like a dildo, a long, slim vibrator, or ben wa balls. After a few weeks of practice you can try adding a specially designed PC-muscle "barbell" to build even more strength. An excellent choice is Nectar Product's Crystal Onyx Vaginal Weight Lifting Egg by San Diego Tantric workshop leader Taylor Lamborne. She designed the Weight Lifting Egg specifically for strengthening PC muscles. The hook at the end of the cord attachment allows weights to be added as you build muscle strength. (Consult the Resources section at the back of the book for information about buying this item.)

Insert your muscle-building object of choice. Squeeze it for three seconds, and then relax for three. Remember: Relaxing the muscles is as important as tightening them, especially if you're prone to tense PC muscles.

With this exercise, be careful not to contract your abdomen, thighs, or buttocks, only your PC muscles. If you feel you're also tightening the other muscles, spend some time in each session trying to isolate and contract the PC muscles without contracting your abdomen or buttocks.

Your goal is to work up to 100 contractions per session, three times a day, five days a week, until you can snugly hold your finger. Might as well go for the burn, girls!

If you can't manage that amount of repetition, it's better to do a few dozen a day than none at all. Develop good PC habits by squeezing and relaxing your muscles, without the barbell, while driving, standing in line, or listening to music. Also, dancing, especially African dance, belly dance, and striptease, exercises the PC muscles, as do masturbation and sex.

Exercise for Tense PC Muscles

To loosen a tense vaginal opening, apply what I call the "Lock Release": With your finger, push down on the PC muscles at the opening of the vagina in the direction of the anus. Do this several times throughout the day. Also, at least three times per week, for one month, massage the band of PC muscles located deep inside the vagina with your finger. Slowly decrease the frequency of the massage over a three-month period, as you notice your muscles becoming more pliable.

Visualization can also help relax tense PC muscles. Lie back and take a deep breath. On the exhale, visually send the breath, along with a verbal command to relax, to your PC muscles. Do this five times. Take note of any sensations you may feel. Do this once a day for three weeks. You will feel the relaxation sensation more fully over time, and often the dull ache of arousal will begin to become noticeable.

Herbal lubricant can make all of these exercises easier, helping to tone PC muscles and encourage a healthy vaginal environment. With the assistance of herbalist colleagues, I have created an herbal lubricant that is available on my website. (Consult the Resources section at the back of this book.)

☽ Tuning In to Your Menstrual Cycle ☾

Ejaculation is easier on some days of your menstrual cycle than others, so select the optimum phase of your menstrual cycle to begin trying to ejaculate.

CHECKING UNDER THE HOOD: MENSTRUAL CYCLE GUIDELINES

Usually, ejaculation is easiest during the twelve days before your period and during your period. It may be difficult to ejaculate if you have just finished your period, and therefore it is best to wait a few days.

> *Menopause:* If you are in perimenopause and your periods are still fairly regular, the same rules apply. If your periods are becoming irregular or stop for months at a time, attempt this exercise at any time, but know, if you are unable to ejaculate, that it may simply be the wrong time of your changing cycle. If your periods have stopped and you are finished with menopause, you get to try this exercise any old time you want! There may be a decrease in the quantity of ejaculate during or after menopause, but more information is still needed about the hormonal nature of the female prostate. Rest assured that your ejaculate will not disappear altogether because of menopause.

> *Pregnancy:* If you are pregnant, ejaculation may be easier than usual, and certainly is not harmful.

> *Birth Control:* It is unknown whether the regulation of your natural hormone levels by birth control pills affects ejaculation in any way, so users should apply the twelve-day rule described above. If you use a diaphragm, know that its pressure on the urethral canal can block the passage of the ejaculate to the outside of the body: You should remove it before practice sessions.

By now you should have a good idea of your "ejaculation readiness." If your result from the attitude-test was a "green light" or "proceed with caution," your muscles are neither overly tense nor overly weak, and you are in an advantageous time of your menstrual cycle, continue to the next section and through to the steps for ejaculation. If your scores were low or you are not in a favorable time in your menstrual cycle to ejaculate, exercise your muscles for a few weeks and continue on to the next section, but do not attempt the steps for ejaculation yet. Now, let's go find the G-spot!

⑤ Techniques for Learning to Ejaculate ⑥
Without an Orgasm

An effective way to begin ejaculating is by manually stimulating your G-spot, without trying to achieve an orgasm. This practical, solo method allows you to get comfortable with the feeling of ejaculating without the pressure to perform with a partner, and without adding the element of orgasm. The method may not seem very erotic, but it is effective for simply experiencing what it is like to ejaculate and for instilling confidence that ejaculation is possible for you.

Therefore, the explorations detailed in this chapter are to be performed alone, before a woman introduces her partner into the process. After you have achieved female ejaculation in this manner, you will have more success ejaculating with a partner. (Ideas and explorations for couples are discussed in Chapter 6.) I recommend this method for a woman's first attempts at ejaculating, as it offers a very good grounding in finding the G-spot, stimulating it, building ejaculate fluid, and expelling it. Taking notice of these sensations, you will begin to make an "erotic map," a mental image of the erotic sites on your body. This erotic map will aid you in communicating G-spot and female ejaculation techniques to your partner. If you follow the steps in each of the next three sections, and master each one before going on to the next, your chances of ejaculating are promising.

GUIDELINES FOR SOLO EJACULATION EXPLORATIONS

The Three Ps—Patience, Persistence, and Privacy

   Patience—New techniques require patience. The first time you made love or touched your clitoris may have felt good, but probably you were unsure exactly how to build this pleasure into an orgasm. The same is true for learning to stimulate your G-spot and to ejaculate. Give it time and allow experience to develop your skill. Enjoy each stage of growth, and don't worry about the "grand finale."

   Persistence—Build skill through persistent practice. Repeat each of the explorations outlined in this chapter three to five times. Each time, your awareness of your G-spot will grow, as you discover areas of pleasure and develop expertise in building and expelling ejaculate. If you don't succeed after you have tried these exercises at least five times, don't despair. Continue to practice with patience. Above all, be kind and encouraging to yourself.

Privacy—Promote success by protecting your privacy. I strongly recommend that women learn to ejaculate without their partners at first. Do not report results to your partner if you have any reservations about doing so. The first few ejaculation experiments are a delicate and vulnerable self-exploration, and they deserve the protection of privacy. Create a safe emotional space in which to practice by realizing that you are not yet in a position to open up erotically with your G-spot. Soon you will be able to share with your partner with greater strength and confidence.

If you describe what you're practicing to your partner, remember that such descriptions are highly erotic to most people. Their excitement can get the better of them and cause you to feel pressured, which can interfere with your budding explorations. Protect yourself with strong and healthy boundaries, by telling him or her that you will share your new knowledge and that it will be very exciting, but only when you are ready.

The Three Ss—Style, Smile, and Sex It Up

Style—Apply your own style and rhythm to every step. Apply the artist's touch to these steps: Go with your intuition, and go with the flow. Make this an opportunity for creative exploration. Get into your body. Get into your emotions and physical feelings. Each woman has her own style and tastes. Let out who you are sexually. Express what you really like and want. Jot down your ideas and use them as guideposts and goals.

Smile—Laugh at ejaculation. Right now, stop reading for a moment, think of ejaculation, and laugh. Whenever you become frustrated, embarrassed, lethargic, or "gyno-deadened" from too much probing, remember that these are only perceptions and you can change them in an instant. Step back and laugh at the scene you are creating. Ejaculating is freeing and joyous—and funny.

Sex It Up—Make these explorations playful and sexy. The techniques described below are straightforward, but they should also feel some-what erotic and create some arousal. They require that you touch and delve into your vagina with relish and abandon. If you have not yet attained that level of comfort with your body, or are not yet familiar with what kinds of physical, mental, and emotional stimulation turn you on, use these explorations to start you on this important journey toward your sexual self. If you still feel uncomfortable or are unsure about what might help you, take some time to think about it and to experiment. (Ask the trained store clerks or mail-order personnel at the sexuality shops listed in the Resources section about books that may help you.) Then try the steps again later.

The Three Rs—Relax, Relax, and Relax!

Relax—Exchange tension for relaxation. Tensing our bodies to build erotic sensations is common when we're trying to achieve orgasm. But tension is also the greatest cause of G-spot numbing and of the inability to let go and ejaculate. Since people tend to cling to "tried-and-true" sexual methods like they do a well-worn blanket, learning to relax during erotic stimulation requires that you replace old habits with new ones. Changing habits takes practice, steady effort, and commitment. But hey, you can do it!

Relax—Build sensation through relaxation and breath. The breath builds sensation and carries erotic energy throughout the body, allowing us to experience the depths of pleasure and emotion that await us in our G-spots. By relaxing and taking deep, slow breaths instead of tensing up, we allow freer circulation, which in turn heightens sensual feelings, which in turn stimulates arousal and ejaculation. In these explorations and whenever you are being sexual, check periodically to see if you are holding your breath. If so, relax, and breathe slowly and deeply.

Relax—Make relaxation second nature. Remembering to relax and breathe during all the explorations is crucial to becoming aware of the G-spot's sensitivity and identifying the feeling of ejaculate building in your body. A few missed orgasms and frustrated nights will probably occur, but this won't go on forever. By the time you have learned to ejaculate, all these new techniques will have become second nature.

SETTING THE STAGE

Create a beautiful space that honors this first attempt at awakening your G-spot. It should be in an environment that is relaxing, private, and personalized for the occasion. Schedule your exploration so that you'll have uninterrupted and extended privacy. If you have extra time, take a relaxing bath. Spread a thick blanket or a few towels on the floor, and place them against something you can lean back on, like the foot of the bed, a wall, or a large dresser or chair. Take a minute to use the bathroom.

Get a large mirror and prop it up in front of you. Set your sex toy and some lubricant nearby and have a box of *white* tissue handy. Remove all your clothes and put on a robe that is loose and opens down the front. Play some soothing music and turn down the lights. Light some incense or scented candles and bring in some flowers, if you'd like.

Now that you are comfortable, it's time to find the G-spot. These next eight steps will build your visual and physical awareness of your G-spot. They will help you to create a mental image of your G-spot and to feel comfortable as you locate and then touch it.

Front View of the G-Spot

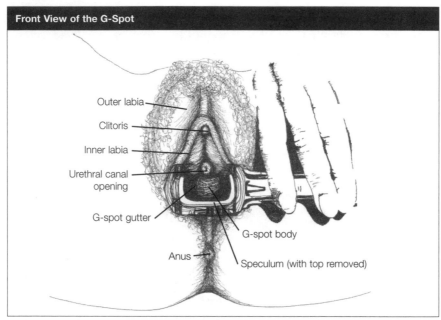

Outer labia
Clitoris
Inner labia
Urethral canal opening
G-spot gutter
Anus
G-spot body
Speculum (with top removed)

Moti Melchizedek

Side View of the G-Spot

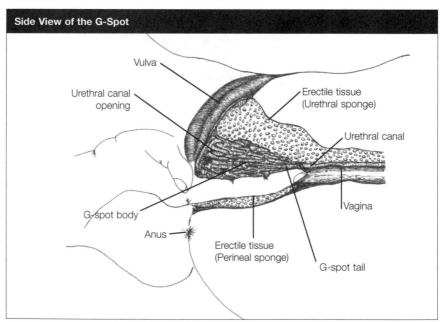

Vulva
Urethral canal opening
Erectile tissue (Urethral sponge)
Urethral canal
G-spot body
Anus
Vagina
Erectile tissue (Perineal sponge)
G-spot tail

Moti Melchizedek

FINDING YOUR G-SPOT

As we discussed in Chapter 2, the erectile tissues that surround the urethra house the female prostate, the G-spot. The area felt through the upper wall of the vagina where the G-spot nestles and protrudes is subtly ridged.

> *Step One—Locate the three central areas of your sex organ.* Sit down on the towel and pull the mirror close. Locate your clitoris and determine how far it is from your vaginal opening by measuring it in finger widths. Some women's clitorises are three finger widths from their vaginal opening, while others are closer. Next, locate your urethral opening and measure how far it is from your clitoris, and then how far it is from your vaginal opening. This helps you get a good picture of how the visible portion of your sex organ is laid out. It also gives you a rough estimate of how much clitoral stimulation you are likely to receive with penetration, and whether your urethral opening will recede into the vaginal opening during penetration, which is the case for many women.

> *Step Two—Observe how your urethra moves.* Next, take a sex toy and lube it up. Insert it into the vagina and watch to see if your urethral opening moves and what it does. If it disappears or comes very close to the sex toy when you push the sex toy in, chances are very good you will not be able to ejaculate with something of substantial size in your vagina (like a penis or dildo or even a finger), even once you are experienced at ejaculating. Change the angle of the sex toy and notice if your urethra behaves differently. If it is one finger width away from the sex toy, you may have an easier time ejaculating with something in your vagina. Even so, the pressure on your urethral canal caused by something in your vagina may cause the ejaculate to be entirely or partially blocked. The purpose of doing this is to get a general idea of how your urethra may behave during penetration, and how blocked or unblocked your ejaculate flow may become during penetration.

> *Step Three—Feel your urethral areas.* Remove your sex toy from your vagina and place it nearby. With your finger, touch your urethral

opening and the spongy area (approximately one-half inch across) that surrounds it. Slide your finger slowly from there into the vagina, about one finger joint deep, pressing gently upward. See how connected your urethra is to your vagina, how it moves, and how soft it is! Notice whatever physical sensations you may feel, perhaps the sensation of needing to urinate.

Step Four—Find the ridges of your G-spot. Slide your finger another finger joint inside. See if you can feel the little ridges of your G-spot, including the one that is the female equivalent of the rim on the head of a penis! They may seem tiny and delicate at first, and can easily be passed over for just a fold of skin. Run your finger from side to side over these ridges for a while. Get to know it. Feel the sensation. Does it remind you of having to pee? Relax into this feeling. This has nothing to do with having to pee; in fact, it's usually the case that when women and men are aroused, they are unable to urinate. Rather, these are the erotic sensations of your G-spot. Get to know these sensations. Visualize your vagina's opening growing fuller as you do this. (If you haven't found the ridges and/or rim, that's fine. You will eventually. Move to the next step for now.)

Step Five—Feel the body of your G-spot. Now, with your finger one to two joints inside your vagina, imagine that a spherical egg has pushed itself partially down into your vagina through its roof. Slide your finger to either side of the imaginary egg, feeling the gutters that run along each side of this "egg." Feel the ridges as you slide your finger from one gutter to the other. The "bubble" between the gutters is the body of your G-spot!

Step Six—Feel the G-spot's tail. Move your finger along the ridges and body of the G-spot (not the gutters). Very slowly and minutely, slide toward the cervix, until you feel the tail end of the spherical egg, at approximately three finger joints. Curl your finger around the tail of this egg. The egg may flatten out a bit at the tail. This is the tail end of your G-spot! Your curled finger is now in the "come hither" position.

Step Seven—Explore the G-spot's size and shape. Explore the entire G-spot area again, feeling the ridges of its body, nestling your finger in the gutters on each side of the G-spot's body, and letting your finger curl around its tail. Stay in contact with your G-spot as you draw your finger slowly over the ridges again, and then out of your vagina. Continue out and up to your urethral opening. Run your finger around your urethral opening. See how closely the G-spot and urethra are connected? Get a sense of the size and shape of your G-spot in its unaroused state. (For an illustration of the parts of the G-spot, see page 80.)

Step Eight—Explore how the PC muscles move the G-spot. Lightly insert your finger again, and experiment with squeezing your PC muscles, and then your buttock muscles. Notice how the perineal sponge (the portion of the erectile tissue on the vaginal floor) comes up to squeeze your finger, and/or how the G-spot moves down to squeeze your finger. Remove your finger and squeeze your PC muscles, then your buttock muscles, again. Notice how the perineal sponge can apply quite a bit of pressure to the G-spot and vice versa. Using a couple of fingers, spread your labial lips quite far apart, so that you can see your vaginal opening clearly. Push your PC muscles forward. In most women, the G-spot moves forward enough that its ridges are visible at the vaginal opening. Isn't it beautiful?

Good! You have not only found your G-spot, but you have explored it to a significant degree and have begun to build your erotic map! Take a breather, then continue on to the next section.

STIMULATING YOUR G-SPOT

The following seven steps will help you get to know the sensitivity of your G-spot and learn how and where to touch it to create the feelings of greatest pleasure. These pleasurable places will form your "erotic map." The stimulation explorations in this section will arouse erotic feelings and cause your G-spot to swell. Therefore, relax into them and try to make them as sexually arousing as possible.

Step One—Create perceptual awareness of your G-spot. Now that you have located and felt your G-spot, you are ready to change the mental view you may have of your vagina. Usually women think of the vagina as a pink, moist cave. Now that cave holds something very significant under its roof! Visualize your vagina becoming warm, wet, and aroused, and your G-spot becoming swollen, while you squeeze and relax your PC muscles. Breathe deeply and relax, feeling in no hurry whatsoever. Lightly tease and stroke your vulva, clitoris, urethra, and vaginal opening as you visualize your swelling G-spot.

Step Two—Squeeze and roll the G-spot between your fingers. Using lube if you'd like, insert a moistened finger along each gutter of the G-spot, going as deep as is comfortable. Breathe in and out and relax. Squeeze the G-spot between your fingers. Roll it around between your fingers as you would your clitoris. It's okay to squeeze it gently but firmly. These touches stimulate the prostate gland to create the ejaculate fluid.

Step Three—Apply gentle, firm pressure. Press all around your G-spot—its body, gutters, tail, and its ridges—moving slowly and minutely. Notice what you feel, and distinguish between pressure (which you might think of as numbness) and sensation (erotic, pleasurable, or even painful feeling).

Step Four—Notice the type of sensation. In the areas that feel erotic, pleasurable, or painful, notice the strength and extent of those sensations. Also notice if you feel a sensation of having to pee, and notice whether that sense is fleeting. If it quickly vanishes, you have probably tensed up. Breathe and relax, and then see if it returns, or if it returns to a different area, or changes into a different type of sensation, perhaps a pleasurable one.

Step Five—Rub and stimulate the G-spot. Keep the pressure firm and begin to make slow, circular movements with your finger. Spend some time on this, and notice whether your G-spot is harder or larger than when you first began this step.

Step Six—Build erotic arousal through stimulation. Continue to press, squeeze, rub, and massage every area of your G-spot. Use different degrees of pressure. Create as much erotic arousal as possible. Build the physical feeling of a full, ripe G-spot by exploring, touching, and rubbing it slowly. Remember to relax and breathe.

Step Seven—Build erotic arousal through visualization. Lay your head back and relax into the sensations of pleasure. Listen to the music and enjoy the quiet of the room, the feel of your vagina, and the sound of your breath. Keep your vagina relaxed and open. Focus all of your attention on the pleasurable sensations of your G-spot. Open your body, mind, and heart to vulnerability and receptivity. Feel the mental, emotional, and physical pleasure of a warm, open, and receptive vagina full of juicy, erotic desire. Use your voice and express these pleasurable feelings.

That was nice, huh? If your G-spot has swollen and you feel physically aroused, you have successfully figured out this area of your erotic map. Proceed to the next section. Otherwise, repeat the two previous exploration sections a few times, until you feel ready to attempt to ejaculate.

For this next set of ejaculation explorations, we need to set aside the mental arousal, but maintain the physical arousal. Things may get a little hectic with these nine steps. Begin by lying on your back.

EJACULATE—LET GO AND LET IT FLOW!

Step One—Build an engorged and swollen G-spot. Increase the G-spot stimulation. Build to a level of arousal at which you feel closer to the urge to orgasm. Notice that your vagina balloons outward and that the body of your G-spot flattens, its tail end nearly disappearing into the roof of the vagina, while near the vaginal opening it grows quite full. The G-spot's ridges, subtle and even unnoticeable at first, become more apparent. Do you feel how very swollen your G-spot is? Welcome this swelling and fullness, and keep stimulating!

Step Two—Notice the shooting "ejaculation rockets." As you stimulate your G-spot, you'll feel sensations of needing to urinate. This is an ejaculation response. A second ejaculation sensation may arise—a subtle streak of pleasure that shoots down your thighs, possibly to your feet. Mild at first, these shooting "ejac rockets," as I call them, can get stronger as you progress to ejaculation. The best way to feel them and increase their sensation is to let them come on their own. Do not try to create them. Instead, relax and enjoy your feelings of arousal. Forgetting about the shooting sensations allows them to occur. Practice stimulating and relaxing until the ejac rockets occur a few times. If they do not occur, that's fine. They may eventually, and they are not necessary for ejaculation. Continue to the next step.

Step Three—Practice pushing out the ejaculate. Keep your finger in your vagina. Stimulate your G-spot as you raise your buttocks off the floor and firmly push outward with your PC muscles as if forcing yourself to pee. Hold a few seconds, then stop pushing but keep stimulating your G-spot. After a minute or two, push, hold, relax, and continue to stimulate. Remember to keep your finger in your vagina the entire time. Repeat this "stimulate-push-hold-relax-stimulate" procedure a few times. Notice, incidentally, if the ejaculation rockets appear or increase in intensity. Your G-spot should feel quite hard and swollen now.

Step Four—Determine your ejaculation readiness. Continue to stimulate to a point where you are so aroused that you crave an orgasm and wish to switch over to your usual method of climaxing. Then ask yourself whether these three statements are true: 1) you feel quite aroused and excited; 2) when pushing, it feels like trying to pee; and 3) your G-spot feels swollen and/or very firm. If the answer to all three is yes, this indicates you are ready to ejaculate. Continue to the next step. Otherwise, go back to step three. If at any point you feel yourself getting distracted or pressured to ejaculate, you can go back to Step Seven of the previous section, relax, and arouse yourself again.

Step Five—Push out the ejaculate while lying down. Take your finger out of your vagina, and immediately push out your ejaculate as if forcing yourself to pee, just like you did in Step Three. Visualize the ejaculate coming out of your urethra. Don't push to clamp down; push to release. This push should be forceful and held for a beat or two. Keep pushing out the ejaculate. You may feel like you are peeing, but you are not. Whether you are successful or not, continue to stimulate and go to the next step.

Step Six—Experiment with another position. Stand up and bend forward slightly, supporting yourself with your free arm. Continue to stimulate your G-spot for a short time. Then take your finger out of your vagina and push. Resist thinking that you are peeing, and keep pushing until all the liquid is expelled. If you're still not successful, stimulate again, try a different position—for example, raised up on your knees, or on your knees while resting on one arm, or squatting. Then, stimulate again, remove your finger, and push out your ejaculate.

Step Seven—Push out another batch of ejaculate. After you ejaculate, without delay, push again right away and a second batch of liquid may be expelled. Extend the pushing effort for as long as the liquid comes out. Your urethra relaxes more, causing you to feel as if, this time, you truly are just peeing. That's okay: You're not. It feels this way because it's likely you are releasing more easily than before and allowing all the fluid out. This is not a time to feel demure or squeamish about splashing all over the place. Let it rip! Push again, or stimulate a little while longer and then push again, and a third round of ejaculate may appear, depending on how aroused you were able to make your G-spot or on how full your G-spot is able to get at this first stage of ejaculating.

Step Eight—Examine the ejaculate thoroughly. Collect as much of the ejaculate as you can in the palm of your hand, wiping it from your body, the towel, robe, rug, or wherever it went. Smell it. Look at it. Take a piece of white tissue and pat your vulva with it. Smell that, too. Look very closely at the color.

Step Nine—Go the bathroom and urinate. Take the tissue with you, and bring an unused one. Sit down and urinate. Pat the urine from your vulva and pubic hair. Look closely at the color on the tissue. Smell it. Now, compare it to the tissue you used to blot up the ejaculate.

If the first one shows a clear stain and has no smell, and the other is faintly yellow-tinged and smells distinctly of urine....

CONGRATULATIONS! YOU EJACULATED!

The proof is right in front of you. Amazing, isn't it? Enjoy the excitement! Tell your girlfriends and go out and celebrate. Regardless of your age, you have made yet another true passage into womanhood.

If you cannot tell the difference in the tissue test, or if it looks and/or smells as if your ejaculate has some urine in it, don't worry about it and read the sidebar "I Think I Peed!" (see page 89). Unless you did not arouse your G-spot, it is very likely you still ejaculated, so congratulate yourself!

⊙ Distinguishing Between Ejaculation ⊙ Sensations and the Urge to Pee!

For many women, the urge to ejaculate feels just like the urge to pee or like an urge that can rocket all the way down the legs ("ejaculation rockets").

Sometimes when I make love, I'll notice a third sensation, a type of "shooting" in my lower abdomen. This is not like the ejaculation rockets, where the sensation rockets down the legs, but more subtle. Initially, all the ejaculation sensations took me by surprise, but over the years they have grown into pleasant and rather exciting signals that

~ *I Think I Peed!* ~

It is highly unlikely that you will pee when you practice these steps to learn how to ejaculate without an orgasm. But if you do, or if you smell a faint odor of urine, here are some reasons why that may have occurred:

1. You have not properly aroused your G-spot. Repeat the section: "Stimulate Your G-Spot."

2. You may be in a phase in your monthly cycle where your ejaculate feels heavy and salty, or your ejaculate may be tinged with urine. Remember that there are trace amounts of urine in female ejaculate, and in some phases of your monthly cycle the smell of urine can be more pronounced. Do not worry about it if this occurs, but notice if your ejaculate smells less like urine during a different time in your menstrual cycle.

3. You may be one of the few women who can pee when your G-spot is aroused and full of ejaculate, like some men can pee when they are aroused and their penises are hard. Do not worry about it. Continue to practice ejaculating and experimenting with distinguishing between the sensations of urination and the sensations of ejaculation.

4. If you find the fear of peeing is stopping you from ejaculating, read the following sidebar "Dealing with the Fear of Peeing" (ooo page 00).

my G-spot is warming up, the ejaculate is moving, and my body is preparing to ejaculate.

Some women experience a fourth ejaculation sensation which is often confused with a urination sensation, a burning feeling like that associated with infections and irritation. Dr. Shannon Bell, Ph.D., calls this sensation the "liquid fire" of ejaculation.

It may be difficult to believe that these sensations—whether burning feelings, chill-like tingles up and down the legs, subtle shooting sensations in the pelvis, or just that "pee urge"—could be anything *but* signals of needing to pee or worse, of illness. But guess what? In the context of G-spot arousal, these sensations, and probably others, are signs that ejaculation is knocking on the door.

A woman from the G-spot chat group describes her budding ability to distinguish between signs of ejaculation and signs of urination:

> In the six months since I began experiencing FE, when I masturbate I notice an interesting sensation, in what I can only guess is my urethra, during clitoral orgasm. It's almost like the "pee-hole" is spasming a bit and I have a feeling that means my body is trying to overcome its habit of avoiding urinating anywhere besides the loo. It's an interesting sensation.

~ Dealing with the Fear of Peeing ~

Distinguishing between the pee urge and the ejaculate urge can be tricky. If you feel the fear of peeing may be keeping you from ejaculating, one way to sidestep having to differentiate between the two is to go to the bathroom before you attempt to ejaculate.

Another way to let go of the fear of peeing while trying to ejaculate is to face up to the possibility of peeing. Do not be afraid to pee in your experiments. In fact, prepare your exploratory space as if you were going to have to wipe up urine! It's not a big deal to pee in this context of exploring your body. The chances are very high that you will not pee, but if the thought of doing so during these experiments repulses you, consider how much you fear peeing, and how difficult it may be for you to *let go* into ejaculating.

The simplest way to sidestep the fear of peeing is to trust your body. If you followed the steps and felt your G-spot swell with ejaculate as you stimulated it, trust that the ejaculate will come out. Let go and let it flow! As you become comfortable with ejaculating, you will develop more awareness of the subtle variations in the urge to ejaculate. Relax into these urges. Welcome ejaculation's surprising insistence.

Learning to reinterpret bodily sensations and develop new perceptions can take time. For years I avoided touching my urethral opening at all costs, because of the severe pain and chronic frequency of my bladder infections. I fiercely protected it from my partner's touch, too. It took me many years to even consider that this area could be erotic. Now the irritation I have lived with for most of my sexual life is much improved and, in fact, my urethra feels soothed by my ejaculate.

When you become aware of the movement of your ejaculate inside your body, you become tuned in to your urges to ejaculate. You may be delighted to discover how often you feel the urge to ejaculate, and be surprised by its urgency and insistence. Unlike the tension response triggered by the urge to urinate, in which the urethra tenses in order to hold back the urine stream, you can relax into the pleasurable feelings of the ejaculate urge. You may even come to miss it on days when it is absent, for whatever reason.

Now that you have ejaculated, you probably feel excited and ready to try it with your partner, but don't rush into trying ejaculation with another person yet. Keep working on building your erotic map first. You will be able to communicate more clearly to your partner about your G-spot and female ejaculation techniques. Practice ejaculating *with an orgasm* by yourself first, as explained in the next chapter. If you have never successfully masturbated to orgasm, begin your first attempts at an orgasm by using the explorations that I described above. You'll be one of the lucky few who get to start your erotic journey with an understanding of the G-spot and female ejaculation.

CHAPTER FIVE

Ejaculate with an Orgasm

◆

Jessica found the stories about women ejaculating far-fetched, but she could also sense her body wanted some sort of release. She considered this for a while, gradually warmed up to the idea of women ejaculating, and finally decided to give it a try.

She sat down one wintry evening in front of a crackling fire and unwrapped the sex toy she had purchased in San Francisco. She slid it into her vagina and lay back to feel the sensations of her G-spot. She was quite surprised at the immediate jolt of pleasure she felt. The strong sensations initially struck her as strange and made her want to stop stimulating her G-spot, but she forged ahead, continuing to stimulate herself to see where her body would lead her.

Just as she was on the edge of orgasm, a gentle stream of fluid seemed to flood the rug beneath her. She stared at the puddle silently as she recovered from her orgasm, more surprised by the incredible longings that had arisen in her heart. She felt almost overwhelmed with a desire to be close to a partner, to share the sensuous pleasure of the fire and the crystalline feel of the dimly lit room. Her body felt luxuriously relaxed, and she lay back next to her neglected puddle of ejaculate and dreamed about the man she'd like to have come into her life.

The steps detailed in the last chapter for learning how to ejaculate may have seemed lacking in erotic appeal. These non-orgasmic explorations are useful for getting this enchanting female fountain unsealed and proudly spouting again. Now the fun begins, as you get to use what you learned and integrate it into your sex life, making it a natural part of your orgasmic celebrations.

In this chapter, we'll begin by exploring the three types of orgasms. Then we'll explore techniques for ejaculating with each type of orgasm. The chapter also looks at some G-spot sex toys, suggests ways of recording your experiences and progress, and discusses methods for dealing with the emotions and longings that G-spot orgasms can trigger.

Every woman's experience, both physical and emotional, of a G-spot-related orgasm is unique. As we explore your orgasms and how they work with female ejaculation, use the definitions provided here as guideposts only. Not enough experience by ejaculating women has been collected to make absolute statements, and absolute statements should never be made about orgasm anyway. As guides, however, these definitions will be helpful in sorting out the confusion that exists about what G-spot orgasms are and how they relate to female ejaculation.

☉ Three Kinds of Orgasms ☉

In Chapter 2, in the section on "Orgasms and Female Ejaculation," we mentioned the nearly exclusive focus on clitoral orgasm since the 1950s. Sexologists Irving and Josephine Singer addressed this imbalance by identifying three types of female orgasm, two of which do not involve direct clitoral stimulation.

Clitoral (vulvic) orgasms involve rhythmic contractions of the PC muscles, feel insatiable, and can be achieved without penetration. Heavy panting is the type of breathing that occurs with a clitoral orgasm.

Uterine (vaginal) orgasms are deeply emotional and satisfying, and take place only if something, such as a penis, dildo, or fingers, is in contact with the cervix. Strong, deep, quick thrusting jostles the uterus and stimulates the sensitive peritoneal membrane, which lines and protects the organs of the abdomen and pelvic area. These orgasms do not involve the rhythmic contractions of the PC muscles. Breathing is suspended (the apnea response) for twenty to thirty seconds just prior to sexual climax.

The blended (G-spot) orgasm involves a combination of clitoral and uterine stimulation and has characteristics of both types of orgasms, including the uterine orgasm's emotional involvement and the clitoral orgasm's PC muscle contractions. The breathing suspension (apnea response) is brief and repetitive. Suction of the cervix/uterus occurs with this orgasm, as well as a pronounced "tonic" feeling from relaxation of the deep vaginal (uterine) muscles. (For more details on these types of orgasms, see Chapter 2, "Orgasms and Female Ejaculation.")

In *The Golden Notebook*, author Doris Lessing described the "vaginal" orgasm as "so complete that subsequent climaxes are quite impossible for at least a day." She believes the release of tension from this type of orgasm is akin to that experienced from a good cry. In classic feminist style, she monitored her facial expressions during a clitoral orgasm and a G-spot orgasm. She noticed her teeth were bared and her brow was furrowed during the clitoral orgasm, whereas during the G-spot orgasm her brow was smooth and the corners of her lips were drawn back.

Although there may be other ways to orgasm and other methods to explore, the focus of this chapter is on understanding how these three orgasms work with female ejaculation. Therefore, the terms that I've chosen to use in this book for these three orgasms are: a clitoral orgasm (vulva), a uterine orgasm, and a G-spot orgasm (blended or vaginal).

These three types of orgasms are not separate and distinct activities or experiences. Imagine a continuum, or spectrum, that covers all three kinds of orgasm. Women who experience orgasms *exclusively from clitoral stimulation* are at one end, and those who achieve orgasms *exclusively from deep vaginal penetration* are at the other. Most women, who experience various combinations of these two types of orgasms, fall somewhere in between and have G-spot orgasms.

Since the G-spot orgasm takes up the bulk of the continuum, chances are good you have already experienced a G-spot orgasm. To help determine where on the continuum your G-spot orgasm is occurring—closer to the clitoral orgasm or the uterine orgasm, read the statements about technique below and choose the one that *most often* applies to you:

⚬ I have an orgasm only with clitoral stimulation. Score 1

⚬ I orgasm primarily from clitoral stimulation with some vaginal penetration. Score 2

❧ I use penetration and clitoral stimulation equally to achieve orgasm. Score 3

❧ I orgasm primarily from penetration, with some clitoral stimulation to achieve orgasm. Score 4

❧ I orgasm through deep penetration and thrusting only. Score 5

SCORE: **1:** Clitoral Orgasm   **2–4:** G-Spot Orgasm   **5:** Uterine Orgasm

Spectrum of Clitoral, G-Spot, and Uterine Orgasms

1	clitoral stimulation only
2	clitoral stimulation primarily with some vaginal penetration
3	penetration and clitoral stimulation equally
4	penetration primarily with indirect clitoral stimulation
5	deep penetration and thrusting only

Clitoral Orgasm ——— G-Spot Orgasm ——— Uterine Orgasm

Deborah Sundahl

The more your answers fall into the middle of the spectrum, the more your PC muscles come into play and the better your chances are of ejaculating during your orgasm. Therefore, for your first attempts at ejaculating with an orgasm, you'll achieve the most success if you are having a G-spot orgasm. As you get more practice with ejaculating during sexual interaction and orgasm, you'll be able to ejaculate just about anywhere on this spectrum of orgasms.

This orgasm spectrum should not be taken to imply that the uterine orgasm is the best or most desirable orgasm. All these orgasms are good and satisfying. However, when a woman begins to awaken to the call of her G-spot, she often experiences a growing dissatisfaction with her clitoral orgasms. A woman who wrote to me after visiting my website explains:

> Well, I am now thirty-eight and starting to realize that I have not allowed myself to truly and fully enjoy my orgasms. Most of my orgasms are from clitoral stimulation, using a vibrator. For some reason, I feel unsatisfied and almost disappointed after climaxing. I finally found the G-spot (I think) and was surprised by the pleasure I felt. I am still a bit uncomfortable about it (probably because I don't know exactly what I'm doing) but feel like if I can learn more about it from an expert, then I can not only enjoy the G-spot but also ejaculating. I have heard that women get such pleasure from ejaculating. I feel like I'm missing out on all the fun. My husband is also open to this but doesn't quite understand how it all works.

The spectrum of orgasm is presented to offer you a clearer picture of what type of orgasm you are experiencing, and to provide more precise language with which to differentiate your experiences and communicate them. Many women and men are confused about what types of stimulation are triggering what types of orgasms. Consider this letter from a woman on the G-spot chat group, who was calling her orgasms "clitoral," when they are in fact G-spot, though toward the clitoral end of the spectrum.

> I easily attain ejaculation with clitoral stimulation only. Yes, when I stimulate the tissue around the urethral (opening) head, I have a clitoral orgasm.

As we have learned, the urethra is stimulated by the pelvic nerve, and it is the pelvic nerve that triggers greater PC-muscle activity and aids ejaculation. Note that this woman is stimulating the head of her G-spot—her "urethral opening and surrounding tissue"—not her clitoris.

She continues to explain how she best achieves ejaculation:

> I cannot make myself ejaculate. I have the world's most delicious lover
> and he gets me there many times orally, and also during penetration.
> There's no guarantee ejaculation will happen, although orgasm
> inevitably does.

As shown on the continuum, clitoral stimulation, plus some penetration, is a G-spot orgasm. But because it is so close to the clitoral orgasm, this second G-spot orgasm usually produces only sporadic or unpredictable ejaculation. Consider this observation by Roger, a contributor to the online G-spot chat group:

> My love (and I) can clearly distinguish between clitoral and G-spot-
> initiated orgasms because of the degree of their intensity and the
> difference in sensation. It has been her observation that when she
> masturbates using clitoral stimulation, she has not had a significant
> FE. She has not been able to FE alone. (I guess that makes me special
> to her.) She cannot get her fingers in the right orientation to stimulate
> her G-spot by herself.

This woman most likely masturbates without much penetration and perhaps experiences more penetration and hence more G-spot stimulation with her partner, which explains why she ejaculates with her partner and not when she masturbates alone.

Consider this woman, writing to the chat group, who has moved her G-spot orgasms further down the spectrum, away from the clitoral orgasm end:

> I'm in my forties and have been able to climax/ejaculate through
> clitoral stimulation since my teen years. But it is only since last year
> that I have "learned" how to not only climax through G-spot stimulation
> but also experience the most amazing ejaculations! For whatever
> reason, the fluid I produce is much more copious through G-spot
> climaxes (a demitasse as opposed to a couple of teaspoons).

Without further details on how exactly she masturbated to the "clitoral" orgasms that produced the teaspoons of ejaculate, I am assuming she was unknowingly stimulating her G-spot in some fashion, very likely through stimulation of the tissues that surround the urethral opening. Now, she is obviously stimulating her G-spot more than her clitoris and noticing a difference in her orgasms, as well as an increase in the amount of her ejaculate. Another letter from Roger, on the G-spot chat group, helps to differentiate a strictly clitoral orgasm from a G-spot orgasm:

> I have tried and tried to cause my love to have an FE with oral sex by direct stimulation of the clitoris. Unfortunately, I have not been successful when my tongue is applied to my love's clitoris. However, I have, on two occasions, been able to cause a FE with my tongue stimulating her G-spot. However that is very hard to do—tongue rapidly fatigues! I have observed that if I stimulate her clitoris for an extended period of time, nearly to the point of orgasm, and then try to rub her G-spot, I cannot get the G-spot to enlarge to induce her to FE. I can't seem to get a super dual orgasm.

Roger is giving another example in which a woman does not ejaculate from clitoral stimulation alone. Interestingly, he describes being unable to arouse the G-spot after intense clitoral stimulation. As he puts it, it is too late, by the time she is aroused, to switch from a clitoral to a G-spot orgasm, which would induce ejaculate.

Clitoral stimulation does not prohibit ejaculation *if* it is used equally with G-spot stimulation or as an aid to G-spot orgasm. Roger may be helped by stimulating the clitoris less and applying more direct pressure to his partner's G-spot.

Remember: The clitoris and the G-spot connect to different nerves, and it is the nerve related to the G-spot (the pelvic nerve) that leads to ejaculation. The pudendal nerve is stimulated by the vulva area, including the clitoris, and triggers only the first third of the PC muscles. The majority of the PC muscles and the uterine muscles do not contract during a clitoral orgasm, and as these are the muscles that aid ejaculation, ejaculation does not occur. The contractions of the G-spot-stimulated PC muscles are also more powerful and more noticeable to your lover.

Frank, from the G-spot chat group, notes:

> My love does not have these intense muscle contractions with clitoral
> stimulation. Most of the time, she has intense contractions of the
> pelvic muscles at the time of her FE. Most of the time, my love does
> not ejaculate with great force, but rather gushes.

Paul writes:

> These contractions have been so intense and so strong that she is
> able to expel my erect penis with her ejaculate!

These two men's observations show how G-spot stimulation, strong
muscle contractions, and ejaculation go together. They also illustrate the
many different types of G-spot orgasms that are possible. None, of
course, are better than another. The spectrum is not included here as a
means to create "ejaculating superfemales," as a few sexologists fear, but
rather to help you navigate your G-spot and female ejaculation experiences with more confidence.

Here is a woman, responding to my website, who has G-spot orgasms
that are more to the uterine end of the spectrum, producing a spectrum
score of 4 or 5:

> For me these ejaculations come really whenever I want them to. The
> one thing that works for me is hard pressure in the vagina, like a hard
> pumping action.

Her comment is interesting in that once you become an experienced
ejaculator, it will start to feel to you as if ejaculation can come whenever
you want it to. This is due to many factors, primarily to not unconsciously stopping the flow of ejaculate, and more G-spot stimulation
than clitoral stimulation.

Maureen, a contributor to the G-spot chat group, has reached an ability to have uterine orgasms that some of us can only dream of—or may
prefer not to, as she will explain. Indeed, women may discover a much
greater range of uterine orgasms as they become more adept at G-spot
orgasms and ejaculating, and learn to isolate and activate their uterine

muscles more (as mentioned in Chapter 2). She describes her experience to the G-spot chat group:

> Located deep inside the vagina near the cervix is a soft "button" that swells, then deflates as it emits [ejaculate through the urethra]. It has been referred to many times on this list by me and by others. There is one woman in *The G-Spot* book who says that only a man with long fingers can reach her squirting spot. It is way in there. This orgasm is quite rare and so earth-shattering as to cause nervous breakdowns in some women. Watch the movie *Bliss*.

> I experienced this orgasm as feeling every deep feeling I have ever felt all at once—sort of like the cliché of your life flashing before your eyes at the moment of death. This type of extreme orgasm associated with this spot may not be something most people would want very often, or perhaps at all. I never know when these extreme kinds will sneak up.

> After this first experience with this type of orgasm, I was not in a state of bliss but of shock. I just lay there wide-eyed, too stunned to speak. Lots of kinds of orgasms can be associated with FE.

Remember Doris Lessing's description in Chapter 2 of "vaginal" (G-spot or uterine) orgasms as being "emotion and nothing else"? Or Freud's theory of "vaginal" orgasms being more "mature"? While I prefer Lessing's description of vaginal orgasms to Freud's labeling, it would appear that sexologists in the past centuries missed a big piece of women's sexuality. This is probably because information about the female prostate was missing from the annals of science, and the vast majority of scientists and sexologists were not taking women's experiences of their bodies seriously. This attitude still persists, as shown by an article by Dr. Terry Hines, a male gynecologist, published in the *American Journal of Obstetrics and Gynecology*. Hines' work made the front page of *USA Today* in 2001. The headline? "The G-Spot: A Gynecological UFO?" That's right, and I'd say it just landed.

Now, how to drive this new space ship? It's easy enough. You have already learned where the G-spot is located and how to stimulate it. And now you have a better idea of what type of stimulation you use to achieve your usual orgasm. The type of orgasm will determine the ease or difficulty with which you may ejaculate during orgasm, and how much fluid you can expect.

So let's move on and ejaculate with an orgasm!

⚙ Techniques for Ejaculating with an Orgasm ⚙

If you usually rely only on clitoral stimulation to orgasm, you will not be able to ejaculate during orgasm with any regularity, in any noticeable quantity, or with any ease, and it's very likely you won't be able to ejaculate during orgasm at all. You will have to change your technique only slightly in order to ejaculate, however, so that you are stimulating some part of your G-spot, and therefore your pelvic nerve. In this way, you are sliding yourself a bit down the orgasm spectrum into the G-spot orgasm range.

Turn your clitoral orgasm into a G-spot orgasm. If you use mostly clitoral stimulation to achieve orgasm, spend more time using a G-spot sex toy (discussed later in this chapter) or finger to stimulate your G-spot and develop your G-spot orgasm. Especially if your first attempts to ejaculate were unsuccessful, you have to stimulate your G-spot more before you begin stimulating your clit. Practicing this type of orgasm may take several sessions. Relax, slow down, and feel the sensations, as outlined in Chapter 4. Remember the places you identified on your erotic map when you did the G-spot stimulation explorations, and touch them in the ways that feel best. For these practice sessions, *turn off the vibrator.*

Masturbate more slowly, taking more time to become aroused. Spread the sensations of arousal around your body by breathing deeply and making sure you are relaxed. Forego fantasies in exchange for focusing on the physical feelings.

Move from G-spot orgasm to ejaculation. Now you can try to ejaculate. In order to create a G-spot orgasm instead of a clitoral-only one, continue making small changes in the way you do things. Stimulate the erectile tissue around your urethral opening; now you're involving the G-spot! Get yourself so aroused that you're ready to orgasm. Attempt to ejaculate—using the same pushing technique from Chapter 4—with this orgasm. Continue stimulating the area around your urethral opening or other parts of your G-spot. You can add your vibrator back in, briefly, if you still need it to achieve orgasm. Slowly, though, rely more on fingers, toys, or partner penetration, moving your orgasm farther down the spectrum.

It feels awkward at first for most women to climax this way. Just spend more time stimulating your G-spot and enjoy the sensations. Practice with this new emphasis for a while. You may not be able to have a G-spot orgasm right away and that's okay. In time, you will. For now, take the new skills as far as you are able, then switch to your regular way to have an orgasm, and keep trying to ejaculate.

If you are already using a combination of clitoral stimulation and G-spot stimulation to have an orgasm, your chances for ejaculation are fair to very good. Experiment with your G-spot orgasm to get to know it better. Take your time. Notice how your body feels, notice if you have fantasies or longings. If stimulating your G-spot brings up strong feelings of lethargy, anger, or loss, continue reading this chapter and then go to Chapter 8, which deals with emotional difficulties and blocks that may arise with G-spot awakening.

Moving from G-spot orgasm to ejaculation. This is the time to do whatever you usually do to have an orgasm. Just follow your erotic map, incorporating more of the G-spot sensations, and spend a little more time there. When you do stimulate your clitoris, place a little less emphasis on it and a little more on your G-spot. Be sure to breathe and emote and move your body and do whatever you feel like doing. Build up the ejaculate. Take time to work up to a good orgasm. Do some deep thrusting with your fingers or sex toy at the end, just before your orgasm.

When you feel ready to ejaculate with an orgasm, here are three crucial rules to follow to release those waters:

1. Have your orgasm in the position that you used to successfully ejaculate without an orgasm.

2. Push out just before you reach the apex of your orgasm.

3.   Let the push expel whatever may be in your vagina—such as your finger or a sex toy—a clear pathway for your ejaculate is usually necessary. Timing is essential.

If you wait too long into an orgasm to push, or begin to push too early, you won't ejaculate. If this happens, don't be concerned. It just takes practice. Once you've become an experienced ejaculator, this timing will become automatic and you won't have to think about it. Eventually, your involuntary orgasmic muscle contractions and your practiced ease with "letting go" will take over to push out the ejaculate at precisely the right moment during orgasm.

If you ejaculated with an orgasm, super! CONGRATULATIONS!

If not, you will! Keep trying without pressuring yourself. Remember to laugh if you are getting frustrated and try letting go of your focus on ejaculation for a while. The rest of this chapter offers further help handling the emotions of G-spot awakening and orgasm, and discusses sex toys that stimulate the G-spot in the way that promotes ejaculation.

⊚ Ground the Romance ⊚

If you are having trouble getting used to G-spot stimulation, remember that it is emotional by nature. "Letting go" isn't only about overcoming the fear of urinating, but about letting one's emotions flow as well.

In *Women Who Love Sex*, Gina Ogden, Ph.D., observes that even recent surveys and studies on sex use definitions of sex that don't take into account the full range of women's experiences of sex. She believes most surveys and studies are too technical and analytical, modeled on a male approach to sexual response, therapy, and research. She is certain that "none [of the studies] deal with the complexities of women's sexual relationships or dives deeply into the rich, murky areas of feelings and meanings." She points out that in not one of these surveys were women asked to define what "sex" means to them—an alarming omission. Dr. Ogden goes on to say that very few sexuality researchers, if any, have "ever suggested a continuum of pleasures or a sexual response cycle that is more attuned to women's experience."

Many of the longings and feelings women have about themselves, their relationships, and life in general are erotic at their root, and their physical, sexual home is in a woman's G-spot. If a woman isn't aware of her G-spot and the feelings it holds, the feelings can flounder around in the psyche, causing women to be more detached from their libidos and less easily aroused than they are capable of being. The following simple visualization exercise can help connect the physical and emotional aspects of sex. It offers a way to affirm your emotions and arouse your G-spot at the same time.

How to Ground the Romance. Lie down in a quiet room. Allow all the longings you have in life (OK, maybe just a quarter of them!) to come into your heart and mind and flood over you. Then, picture a big funnel-shaped object over your head that goes down through your heart and into your G-spot.

Sweep all the yearnings into the funnel and see them going into your G-spot. Feel your G-spot become erotically charged. Imagine it getting larger.

Nice, huh? It works.

Repeat this visualization daily, or as often as possible, until you can transfer those romantic foreplay feelings into your G-spot anywhere, at any time, without needing anything but a minute of focused concentration.

This visualization helps you take responsibility for your erotic desires and helps you direct them to your sexual center, where they can function as triggers for your sexual expression, instead of lying around helter-skelter in your mind or being projected onto people who invoke your soulful fantasies but are not, in reality, able to deliver.

When you can ground your soulful and naturally "murky" feminine desires into your physical, sexual center, you no longer need to put the responsibility on your mate to connect your emotional longings to your sexual self. Ground the romance in your G-spot. It's your organ to activate. Once you master this skill, you can meet your man halfway and be a truly equal sexual partner. As Dr. Ogden says, "by taking this kind of power, women may be able to narrow the gender gap."

◉ Women Who Run with the Water ◉

Cultural notions of femininity can create obstacles to women being sexually "wild." Although those ideas have changed radically in the past forty years, the old notions linger, and the changes take time to internalize. Now and then, I still stop myself from experiencing more pleasure or ejaculating more because I feel I may be too wild and will offend my boyfriend. Changing deep-seated attitudes takes time—maybe a lifetime.

Until not too long ago, the socially approved picture of femininity was still a Victorian one: nice, proper, pleasant, neat, and controlled. A woman was expected to have a sweet, quiet, perfect little orgasm while she lay still and didn't sweat. G-spot orgasms and female ejaculation are wild and emotional by nature. They can feel strong, explosive, tumultuous, passionate, large, messy, chaotic, complicated, and curious.

By traditional American standards, female ejaculation is untamed. It can feel too emotional, too unusual, too shocking, and too much like a "bad behavior" that invites rejection. But as Clarissa Pinkola Estes, author of *Women Who Run with the Wolves*, and others have said, the wild side is the residence of the true, soulful self. If you have not allowed yourself to express your erotic wild side, you may be a bit taken aback and ask yourself, "Am I *that* untamed inside?" "Am I *that* hungry, *that* desirous?" The answers are unequivocally "Yes," "*Yes*," and "YES!"

Moving, shaking, moaning, roaring, yipping, screaming, sobbing, laughing, yodeling, pounding, rolling, and gushing are some of the emotional and physical manifestations of the untamed, yet 100 percent female, erotic fountain. You'll feel great after all this messiness. Accept the emotions that will invariably arise with G-spot stimulation and pleasure. If you are:

Angry?	... then ...	**Roar!**
Sad?	... then ...	**Cry!**
Happy?	... then ...	**Laugh!**
Frustrated?	... then ...	**Pump hard!**
Loving?	... then ...	**Be slow and gentle!**
Irritable?	... then ...	**Gush wildly!**

Express yourself! Let emotions and ejaculate flow. Don't be afraid to be a woman who runs with the water (or the wolves!). If you feel irritable, moan and move. Something is in there—yearning, longing, desire—that wants out, and it's not only ejaculate, but emotions and feelings.

At its heart, sexuality is a personal expression, which is why some ancient texts refer to it as an art form. A woman's erotic potential for self-expression is physically located in an awakened G-spot.

Sexual expression ebbs and flows throughout your lifetime. If you learn to listen to its rhythms and signals, it can point the way to growth and change. Sexuality skips around the issues of life, sometimes sending you forward into a new area, or backward to explore an older piece. As one young woman said to me after experiencing the secrets that the G-spot can reveal, "I reconnected with a piece of my sexuality that I had forgot I had lost . . . an 'innocence' and a freedom to be myself that touched me so deeply I feel moved to tears when I think of this new self that is now a part of me again." (See the Resources section for books that can help you explore this transformative power of sexuality.)

Each time you approach sexuality it can be a new experience if you use emotions and expressions as its backbone. Whatever may come up for you, emotionally or physically, mentally, or spiritually, let it flow! Welcome its message or simply enjoy its pleasure.

⊚ A G-Spot and Ejaculation Journal ⊚

Attempting all these new techniques, toys, positions, and adventures with yourself and others offers an overflowing gift bag of opportunities. Such bounty causes a range of emotions and experiences, and your explorations may push buttons that you'll need to take "time outs" from occasionally. A sexual exploration journal is a handy tool for such times. It helps you to remember what transpired the last time you practiced, offers insight into how you might refine your approaches and techniques, and aids in communicating to your partner more clearly what you have learned so far.

Journals are fun to buy. Many are beautiful, and some are even hand-made. The act of purchasing one is nurturing to the self, because taking time for yourself and learning to give voice to things that are important to you floods your body and mind with warmth and relaxation—a comforting and useful frame of mind in which to approach your explorations with your G-spot and ejaculation. The best method for recording your experiences in your journal is to divide each of your entries into six parts: date, activity, emotional response, physical response, old attitudes, and new attitudes. Here's an example:

DAY, DATE, TIME, AND LOCATION: Monday, January 21, 2003. 7:00 p.m. Bedroom.

ACTIVITY: Stimulate Your G-Spot, Step Four from the female ejaculation book, third time I've practiced it. I used the glass sex toy that arrived in the mail from Toys in Babeland.

EMOTIONAL RESPONSE: Initially resisted settling down. Felt excited but also rather embarrassed. John was out for the evening, and I felt guilty that I was hiding this secret from him. Also nervous that he would come home early and come into the room, and that I wouldn't get the chance to try to ejaculate.

PHYSICAL RESPONSE: My body felt much more pleasure this time as I lay back and relaxed. I can visualize my G-spot much better now. When I inserted the toy, I noticed that it seemed too big because I'm used to my fingers. Then I discovered that the lip on the toy rubs against the back of my G-spot. Oh, that felt incredible! I relaxed and went on to Exercise Five.

OLD ATTITUDE: No old feelings came up this time. Well, maybe the guilt that I can't have this pleasure or the time to explore my sexuality without my boyfriend. That my sexuality is something I share, not something that is totally mine.

NEW ATTITUDE: I like using this new sex toy. I like that I have it. Practiced washing it without feeling hurried or guilty. Put it out on the dresser with a note to my boyfriend: "Getting closer. Can't wait to feel you."

Here are a few entries from the journals of some women friends who were kind enough to share them with me:

Jayce... ACTIVITY: Find Your G-Spot. I don't like touching myself, so right away I wasn't feeling comfortable. This felt like a total assignment. But it was easy to do and easy to find that "corrugated" place, took all of thirty seconds. It's right there, at the front of the opening (of the vagina). I thought, "Well, good! Now just find something around the house to stimulate it with." But I didn't. Afterward, it still felt like a total assignment I had to do. Kind of scares me, too.

Karana... ACTIVITY: Experience a G-Spot Orgasm. I was all alone, so there was no one else's pleasure to be preoccupied with. I felt emotionally relieved no one else was there. I felt extremely horny, you know that time right before your period when you get voraciously horny. I lay back in the tub, feeling the sensation of my G-spot and enjoying the sensation of opening up to the pleasure. I took a lot of time for this, the soap, the sensuality, the caress all over my skin. The orgasm was mindblowing. I don't feel like doing this again for a while, because of all the time, effort, and concentration it takes. I just don't have enough time, emotional motivation, or desire.

Meryl... ACTIVITY: Try to Ejaculate. Today I experienced my first ejaculation. It was intense. It was relieving. It left me feeling complete. And I felt some disbelief. Was this there all along? I took a long walk. I felt whole. I felt a new confidence. I walked to see a horse who lives down the road without any other horses around. I carried some apples with me. I looked into his eyes and saw how loneliness is wearing him down. I cried for him. I cried for his longings. I cried for mine.

Angie... ACTIVITY: Ejaculating with a Partner. I was having sex with Jack, and he started rubbing his cock on me just up against my clitoris on the outside—the head of his penis went from vagina to clit and

back again. Felt really good, and I asked him to do it harder, and the
harder the better. I had an awesome orgasm and ejaculated all over. It
soaked everything. He laughed; he liked it a lot. I'm neither here nor
there with the ejaculation, but I sure liked the orgasm! It felt like an
accident. I don't know if I can do it again, but I remember that area
and I think he does, too.

Journals aren't always written; some are books of personal art. Journals
used for drawing are beautiful (just like journals intended for writing), and
they are larger so that you can draw in them. You don't have to be an artist,
because you are drawing your own feelings, for your eyes only. Let your
emotional body take over from your rational mind for a while and see what
comes off your crayons.

Immediately after you have a practice session, make a drawing of it.
Draw whatever comes off your pen—abstract or literal. Use colored pencil,
watercolors, or crayons. If you want, you can buy a large roll of white shelv-
ing or wrapping paper, unroll it on the kitchen floor, and really go at it.
Whatever you create will help you to remember your experience and track
your progress. Note the date, time, location, your emotional and physical
responses, and your old and new attitudes, just as you would in an ordinary
written journal—you can select one or a few words to describe each of
these things and write them on the drawing, such as:

DAY, DATE, TIME, AND LOCATION: Monday, January 21, 2003.
7:00 P.M. Bedroom.

ACTIVITY: Experience Ejaculation

EMOTIONAL RESPONSE: Bored

PHYSICAL RESPONSE: Fiery sparks

OLD ATTITUDE: Uninterested

NEW ATTITUDE: Reserved interest

My friend Anatolia likes to use this type of self-expression and she shared one of her entries with me a few years back. In the middle of a large piece of paper, she had drawn a big circle in black crayon. Out of the circle poured red and black waves. Yellow was drawn over the black lines of the circle, and little bits of blue traced the red and black waves. Long brown tree trunks were on each side, and green was colored over the empty space at the top of the drawing.

She said the drawing expresses her feelings about her first ejaculation experience because it felt like water, grass, and the sun were growing out of a black and angry hole.

Writing and drawing provide creative methods for recording and processing your experiences. Dance and music are examples of other creative outlets that can also assist you in expressing your new experiences, and yoga and martial arts can help you to integrate them into body memory and your subconscious mind.

Some good books to inspire and help you with this self-exploration are *The Artist's Way* by Julia Cameron, *Writing Down the Bones* by Natalie Goldberg, and for expressive dancing, Gabrielle Roth's video *The Wave.*

Taking this kind of time to let artistic self-expression help you discover and unleash your inner wild and wet woman is nurturing and self-affirming. The ejaculation process offers ample opportunities to open a few doors or redecorate some long-neglected rooms in your psyche, and I encourage you to take advantage of it. I'll never forget a comment my son's former girlfriend, Kara, made to me one day about her discovery of her blossoming sexuality. She exuberantly blurted out, "I feel like this is affecting all areas of my life!" Yes, dear. It is.

For young women like Kara, it's a new discovery; for older women, it can help to make sexuality whole once again, or even for the first time. Younger women are a generation ahead of their older sisters in the sexual self-discovery arena, and this fact is worth celebrating. Women of all ages will gain increased self-esteem from their explorations into female ejaculation and the G-spot and its potential to reveal a hidden, sexual self. This erotic literacy of the self, as Dr. Gina Odgen says, "leads to personal integration and rewarding relationships of all sorts."

⊚ G-Spot Sex Toys ⊚

Years ago, I was teaching a three-hour workshop on the G-spot at Good Vibrations, the premier sex toy store in San Francisco. A shy but attentive young woman, Sondra, asked me only one question: Is it okay to use a toy to try to stimulate the G-spot? Behind me was a wall full of dildos and vibrators, each in its own clear Plexiglas display case, an impressive installation of colors and shapes. "Sure," I said to Sondra, and walked over to the toy display.

This particular workshop occurred before the G-spot became popular enough to have toys made specifically for it, so I had to be creative with my selection. Years before, through keen shopping, I had personally obtained a one-of-a-kind, large, pretty, clear Plexiglas dildo with pronounced "veins" on its body and a large lip around the head. It worked like a charm to awaken my G-spot. I scanned the wall for toys that had these G-spot-stimulating elements.

I selected a lavender dildo that looked like a large cock with a very large lip around its head and a pink, spongy dildo that had waves molded into its surface. I also chose a black plastic vibrator to show what *not* to use. I carried them back to the group and we began to talk about which ones would work best, and why.

Toys are useful for the firm, direct, and concentrated stimulation that you need when you are first awakening your G-spot. Many of the G-spot toys vibrate, but although vibration is a successful method to stimulate the clitoris to orgasm, it is not useful for initial attempts at awakening G-spot sensitivity. In many cases, you can turn the vibrator off and still insert the toy into your vagina to stimulate your G-spot. As your G-spot becomes more sensitive over time, you may find you do not need or like the added stimulation that G-spot sex toys provide. You may even find you ejaculate better with partnered sex than with the G-spot toys, as this woman on the G-spot chat group explained:

> I'm pretty well convinced that the added excitement I get from my
> lover is a major contributor to my ability to FE. It's just not as fun when
> I'm alone with my sex toy.

Traditional G-spot toys are curled at one the end in order to stimulate the tail of the G-spot. (However, that "come hither" curl is undergoing some refinement, as we shall see.) Any dildo that has a large lip is good for this purpose as well. A toy that has a wavy body, or one that has a couple of balls embedded in its body, is excellent for stimulating the body of the G-spot. An example of a toy that stimulates both the tail and the body of the G-spot is the Deluxe Crystal Wand, designed and manufactured by San Diego Tantric workshop leader Taylor Lamborne. Her wand has a ball embedded in its elegant, S-shaped, Plexiglas body. Though Plexiglas tends to dry out quickly, lubricant takes care of this minor drawback.

I encourage you to buy sex toys in women's sexuality shops as opposed to in more traditional, male-oriented stores, because the women's shops are committed to quality, aesthetics, ingenuity, and variety in their products, as well as confidentiality in mailing lists and shipping practices. These stores offer money-back guarantees on their products, and friendly, informed sales consultants who will discuss with you the best purchase for your needs. This handful of women's stores scattered across the country has made erotic shopping for women a fun, help-filled, clean, and well-lighted experience. They are on another planet entirely from the seedy adult-sex shops which still predominate in most of the country, though a few of the latter have finally taken a cue from women's sexuality shops. The cottage-industry products that these newer shops carry are often made and tested by women. (Consult the Resources section at the back of the book for a list of these stores, their locations, and contact information. These stores all have websites and mail-order catalogs.)

These days, the selection of G-spot toys is prolific and varied, and some are downright cute. All are identifiable by the "come hither" curl on the end. Some are expensive, but if you follow the easy-care instructions, they should last for years. The following are a few of the best-selling G-spot toys at some of these wonderful stores (most of these toys are sold at most of the stores, not just the store where they are listed here):

Toys in Babeland's hottest-selling item is the Nubby G vibrator ($14–$20; always check direct for the latest prices or special offers). Rachael Venning, cofounder of this chain of stores in Seattle and New

York, says they've "nicknamed it the 'Nubby Genius' because it has just the right curve, and is made of a firm, yet resilient, jelly rubber. Plus, it is great looking—completely translucent—like water, made solid."

Eve's Garden in New York recommends the Tsunami ($23–$26), a pink or blue transparent jelly-rubber item with a flexible curved end that vibrates. This store also recommends the vibrating and rotating Rabbit Habit ($86). It's made of white, transparent jelly rubber that turns to purple on its curled-up end, and sports a purple bunny rabbit at its base. The bunny's job is to stimulate the clitoris. Inside the toy's body are colorful little beads. Their weight shifts as the toy rotates, providing extra stimulation to the body of the G-spot.

Good Vibrations in Berkeley and San Francisco recommends the Crystal Jelly G-Spot Vibe ($20), which comes in a kit along with their book, *The Good Vibrations Guide to the G-Spot*. Another choice is the Turbo Glider ($18), which has a bulbous head and is hard, pink plastic. They also have green and red Dino Vibes in silicon ($55). (Silicon is not porous like the translucent jelly rubber, so toys made of it are more hygienic, but cost more than those made of jelly rubber.)

The staff at Grand Opening! in Boston says their favorite G spot toy is the Gee Egg Vibe ($19), an ivory-colored, tall, thin, hard plastic vibrator with an egg-shaped protrusion at the top. Another favorite is the Aqua G ($22), a waterproof, clear-blue-glitter jelly-rubber vibrator that curves at the end.

My personal favorites are the beautiful and artistic Pyrex glass sex toys created by Asstroknots. Though most of the toys I've already mentioned are artful enough to set out on the dresser, these take the prize. They are handmade by artisans and the design is patented. Because they are glass, they are not porous, like rubber dildos, which tend to be hard to clean and keep odor-free. These are dishwasher-safe and easy to sterilize (by boiling in water). The smooth texture of the glass, its hardness, and the fact that it can be either cooled or heated can make them preferable to the softer, more rubbery feel of jelly rubber or silicon.

The glass is attractive, and it's safe to use in the vagina because the Pyrex is strong. Asstroknots ran the front tire of a Chevy Impala over one of its toys. All that resulted was the toy created dents in the quarter-inch-thick oak board the demonstrators laid it on! These toys are expensive little art objects ($200 to $600), but they are effective and last a lifetime. They remind me of my old and beloved Plexiglas dildo, but they are much improved.

Asstroknots has refined the effectiveness of the G-spot toy by replacing the curved-up end with a ball and embedding a "bag of marbles" in the base to stimulate the clitoris. The "balls at two ends" design means that both the clitoris and the tail end of the G-spot are stimulated and you get a really snug fit. The Asstroknots website states that women scream when they first use these toys, and I had a similar reaction when I stumbled upon the Asstroknots booth a few years ago at a sex toy convention in Las Vegas. When I picked up one of its toys and felt it, I immediately knew what it could do. I turned away from the table and blushed while my primal woman screamed inside! Finally, a beautiful and effective G-spot toy! Yeow! What was that I said about preferring partnered sex?

Toys in Babeland offers a less expensive version called the Archer Wand ($45). It is a bow of clear acrylic with a round knob on either end. "That knob really hits the spot!" says co-owner Rachel Venning.

Erotic performance artist and sexologist Annie Sprinkle recently came up with a variation on the G-spot sex toy design using gemstones. She says:

> I've tried all the G-spot toys, but I invented one of my own, which I like the very best. It's shaped like a fist with the thumb and finger-tips together. I love it because I can put it in my pussy when I'm masturbating, squeeze my PC muscles on it consistently, and it won't slip out! It's called the Love Handle [$200]. It's carved from black marble, and is a "limited edition" designer dildo (each is signed and numbered), and it also functions as an art object that you can place on your coffee table. The coolness of the black marble also stimulates my G-spot nerve endings.

Sex toys are excellent tools to use initially to discover your G-spot and awaken its sensitivity (and they are good for a lifetime of erotic fun and pleasure!). Here is one story about a Toys in Babeland customer about whom Rachel wrote to me:

> I remember a somewhat skeptical but scientifically minded woman came into the store a few years back. She wasn't sure she believed in the G-spot, but wanted to find it if it was there to find. She read the books, watched your *How to Female Ejaculate* video, and embarked on a program of masturbation. She did not ejaculate for the first few weeks, but finally, with the help of the Crystal Wand, she surprised herself by squirting. She told me all about it and also says she can now do it all the time without having to try so hard.

Much can be accomplished if you set out with confidence and an open mind to awaken your G-spot and to ejaculate like the woman above did. I encourage women to take some time to experiment with all the new techniques that were introduced in these last two chapters. Spend time exploring the orgasmic range—and your feelings about it—that the G-spot orgasm makes available to you, and become more proficient at G-spot stimulation and ejaculation. You're bound to see results. G-spot toys are helpful devices to use during this experimentation, too, and I hope you decide to own at least one.

If you have been able to get through Chapters 4 and 5 successfully, I congratulate you! You are now well equipped to forge ahead into ejaculating with your partner! May your waters flow libidinously throughout your lovemaking!

CHAPTER SIX

Ejaculate with a Partner

Janice was relieved to find that her waters could really flow. She was excited to show her husband. She took him into the bedroom and told him she had a special surprise for him. He was eager to see what was in store.

She lay on the bed and removed her panties. She could already feel her G-spot come alive, and this new sensation and the thrill it made her feel aroused her even more. In fact, she felt an eagerness to feel him inside her that she hadn't felt very often in her sexual life. She had to take a deep breath, remembering to slow it down and enjoy the sensations. She was also very excited to see what would happen.

"I need to get really aroused first," she whispered to him, and he gladly took some extra time to stimulate her. "I like this sensation just inside my vagina," she moaned with pleasure and moved so he could understand what stroke it was she meant. Curious and aroused, he took time to play with this area that seemed to give her a lot more pleasure; she realized she had just introduced him to her "erotic map."

When he entered her, it felt so good. "Please stimulate it very slowly," she said in a husky tone. "I can feel you so well." He grew very excited and paid extra attention to how his strokes were exciting her. It amazed her how his attention to her stimulation increased her own G-spot awareness. She played with her clitoris to bring herself to orgasm, and when she did, she pushed out a beautiful little gush of liquid onto his penis and thighs.

He was surprised and pleased and he came really hard from the excitement her ejaculation aroused in him. Afterward, Janice liked how she felt inside and kissed her husband deeply, pleased with their first ejaculation experience.

As I wrote this chapter, the old wedding saying for the bride kept running through my mind,

Something old, something new,
something borrowed, something blue.

The "something new" item you bring to ejaculating with a partner is confidence in your ability to ejaculate, awareness of your body and the sensitivity of your G-spot, and a better sense of the variety of orgasmic pleasure you can experience. The "something old" (tuck it into your corset!) is a well-deserved ribbon that represents all the uncertainty you've gone through, all your stumbling efforts getting your G-spot to work, and turning cumbersome techniques into skill. The "something borrowed" is an evening from Grandfather Time. And as for blue—the color of water—that's your ejaculate, of course!

This chapter discusses how to tell your partner you want to ejaculate with him, and how to explain the contours of your erotic map. Couples can navigate the first night of female ejaculation with greater confidence by learning which sexual positions are best suited to her ejaculating. Tips on how to deal with that shower of feminine water are explained, as well as some good places to ejaculate freely on your "honeymoon."

Your partner will probably be surprised and pleased with the introduction of female ejaculation into your love life. In any case, he will do one of the following things:

1. Change with you.

2. Welcome you. He has been waiting for this!

3. Resist the change.

The next section will help you minimize any problems with numbers one and three, and optimize number two.

⊚ "Honey, I want you so bad, ⊚ I might gush all over you!"

It's a good idea to tell your sex partner beforehand that you ejaculate. It can be shocking, and you don't need any rejection, nor does your partner need to be caught off guard and looking foolish. And if you share the news ahead of time, you can get out the towels, which seems to get men even more excited.

Before telling a man you are ready to ejaculate with him, assess his knowledge and interest in the topic. Be direct. Simply come out and ask him, "Have you heard about female ejaculation?" He may indeed know all about it. However, the question may put him in a tight spot, as he will be unsure if you are asking him if he knows about it in general, or if he's had experience with it. If he knows about it and has never discussed it with you, he may feel he'll have to tell you where he heard about it and may not want to get into that.

Therefore, be ready to sense any hesitation, and quickly add, "I have been reading about it and trying it and I want to try this with you." That takes the pressure off him, but he may still want to know where you have been trying this out and why you haven't told him. (Even if he doesn't ask, it is likely to be on his mind.) Therefore, tell him you've been reading up on it and have been practicing in order to surprise him, but that the book advised that you tell him before trying it together so he wouldn't be *too* surprised.

That should ease his mind and will get his full interest. In fact, he may want to run to bed right away and see what you're talking about. Since you, not he, initiated this conversation, it's up to you to be ready to show him what you're talking about without expecting him to take the lead.

He may not know what to do and will wonder if he has to change his technique entirely, or do anything at all, so as you lead him to the bedroom, tell him, "If I need you to do something different than what you normally do, I'll tell you." That clear communication will allow him to relax. If he has had some experience with female ejaculation, he may just smile. Tell him you aren't sure if you will be able to ejaculate right away, but you'd sure like to try.

Though most guys these days have had little or no experience with female ejaculation, I've yet to meet a guy who doesn't greet it with acceptance and excitement. Guys like the meat and potatoes of sex, as we explain in the next chapter. So, no worries, girls. That's the wonderful part about guys and sex. Men tend to be more open about and ready for sex than women, and most of them have been waiting most of their lives for a woman to come up to them and tell them in a sexy whisper, "I'm going to do something you're really going to like!"

So "do up" this special event! Enjoy your partner's eagerness. You are ready, and you've certainly gotten his interest up, so don't delay! Take him by the hand and show him what's up! Make it fun and sexy! Remember, in all likelihood this will be his first experience with female ejaculation, so make it a pleasant and memorable one. Even if you don't ejaculate successfully, he won't care as long as he knows that it's not because he did something wrong. You both have some exciting times to look forward to.

◔ Using Your Erotic Map ◔

You began learning about your erotic map in Chapters 4 and 5: So far you've identified the points on your G-spot that are pleasurable to you and the types of touch and duration of touch that turn you on. Your erotic mood on any given day shifts these points, types of touch, and orgasmic sensations around, but in general your erotic map is where you like to be touched and how. You don't have to literally explain, or map out, where the places are or what is attached to what. Most men get turned off by being handed a set of instructions. Simply tell your partner in an erotic way what feels good as he explores your body.

When you are ready to show him what you've learned about your G-spot, keep it fast-moving and fun. Ask him to help you find your G-spot, and tell him how it feels different depending on the touch he uses. Let him know you would like to explore the sensations together. Most men are happy to oblige, and not much more need be said. Anita, a friend of mine, had a very easy and successful time showing her partner the new G-spot areas of her erotic map:

I asked my guy, "Will you help me find my G-spot?" He was intrigued, and I went and lay down on the bed. As we progressed, it felt pleasurable and I became aroused. I asked him to do it lighter or harder, and then, "Oh! Oh! Oh! Please remember that place!" It was an exploration for both him and me, one that was playful, erotic, and free of pressure.

From there we progressed into intercourse. Both of us were aware of the new sensations we had found on my G-spot, so we were both adjusting our movements to see if they could be created with his penis. It was not a big deal, but I told him that when he stroked it slowly "right there" and "there," I started to feel that full feeling in my G-spot. Then we went on to the usual way we make love. But as I had an orgasm, I pushed his cock out and ejaculated on him. He loved this! He got excited and came shortly after that.

Anita's approach involved her partner by encouraging a sense of discovery, without losing the thread of their regular sexual behavior. This is a great way to begin with your partner. He is motivated by wanting you to ejaculate and have pleasure, so he will make an attempt each time you make love to become more in tune with what turns you on. Each time you make love is an opportunity to communicate little bits of information: "Oh, that really feels good!" or "Oh, that is getting more and more sensitive!"

~ Something to Remember ~

As with any sexual encounter with a partner, G-spot knowledge and skill levels will improve over time. It's important to enjoy each encounter for what it is and not make ejaculation the full focus and goal.

⊚ The Best Sexual Positions for Ejaculating ⊚

Taking your newfound ejaculation expertise into the bedroom and sharing it with a partner is exciting. As you develop your sensitivity and your ability to ejaculate, you will find that ejaculation is less a matter of technique and positions and more a matter of losing yourself in the sensations of your awakened G-spot and in the act of love itself. But until your sensitivity and skills have developed to that level, trying some specific sexual positions can help you learn to ejaculate, with or without orgasm, during sex with your partner.

Modified Missionary. Lie on your back and put your legs over your partner's shoulders. This is a good position if you need clitoral stimulation in order to orgasm, and it is a nice way to begin to experience building a G-spot orgasm. He'll have a lot of control over stimulating your G-spot, particularly the opening to the vagina, and you can play with your clitoris to have an orgasm. Focus on perceiving the pleasure of your G-spot, and ease up on your usual clitoral stimulation, using it only to keep things moving. Notice how full your G-spot is getting, and keep your arousal slow so you can get the full amount of time you need for G-spot stimulation. When you feel you want to orgasm and your G-spot feels full, push out and ejaculate. You may find a direct target on his chest or face, and he'll like that a lot.

Mouth and Finger, Yum! This oral sex position is good for achieving a G-spot orgasm if you are used to climaxing clitorally, and also great if you need to practice relaxing. Ask your partner not to use the tongue as a vibrator on your clit, but to caress your clitoris, urethra, and vaginal opening with lips and tongue. Slower is better, so you have time to absorb all the sensations and to remember to relax. When you feel aroused, ask him to insert a finger, ever so slowly, and rub your G-spot very slowly but firmly. Suggest that he try the "come hither" motion, that is mimicked by the curl on the sex toys.

Over time, your G-spot will become more easily aroused, and swollen, and less stimulation will be necessary to feel ready for ejaculation.

The point of this position is to relax and allow the sensitivity and pleasure to grow and evolve by shifting your focus bit by bit from clitoris to G-spot, over many lovemaking sessions.

When you feel like ejaculating, have at it and flood your sweetie's mouth.

Face to Face on a Stool. A tall kitchen stool is perfect for communicating and slowly working up to soulful eye-to-eye communication. If you are used to closing your eyes and burying your head in the pillow, you'll find that in this position you are more present and equal. No one's weight is on anyone, you are face-to-face (he's standing and you're sitting), and it's the right height for him. You can easily sit on a towel, the ejaculate will mostly fall on his thighs and cock, and if you do it in the kitchen, wiping off the tile is a snap. You can look down at his cock, and he can get valuable feedback about the types of strokes he is delivering when he sees your face and hears your delighted sounds.

Because this position provides intense stimulation to the G-spot and a clear, direct way to communicate, this is the best position for both of you to learn how to awaken and stimulate your G-spot. Your clitoris can also be easily stimulated. But know that if your G-spot is becoming more sensitive, this position could feel tender or painful or even close down your awakening sensitivity if you allow penetration before you are ready. If you have found that you are the type of woman who needs or likes to ejaculate without something in your vagina, this position will make it difficult to move your pelvis to push him out when you need to ejaculate, although it can be done.

This position is excellent for deep penetration—if the stool is sturdy—and for exploring how deep, penetrating thrusts can trigger the sensations of a uterine orgasm. It's likely that at first you may not have an orgasm and you may not ejaculate, but it's worth it to explore a uterine orgasm.

Standing up from Behind. The fairly common "doggy-style" position, where the woman is on her hands and knees and is entered from behind, is certainly a good way to ejaculate and many have complete success this way. But especially if your PC muscles are lax, I recommend standing up, slightly bent forward. This position puts more pressure on the G-spot than does the traditional doggy-style. Your partner's movements will push forward against your G-spot, and that's exactly what you want for good stimulation and to build ejaculate. Also, it is easy to move your body if you need to push him out to ejaculate.

Standing up is the most common method women employ to first learn how to ejaculate, and this may be just the position for you. I once ejaculated so profusely in this position I felt I just couldn't stop. I was glad I was in the wilderness. Out and out and out it came, and nearly started a small river. I stopped only because it was a little startling, and I was tired. The wilderness is a good place for thundering and letting loose, and for splashing all over as much as you want. The rule for all these positions should be not to let worry about the mess deter you from ejaculating. You can ejaculate outside, on a hardwood floor, on a kitchen floor, in a shower stall, or even on the shag carpet! Heck—why not?

In all these sexual positions, it is important to have your G-spot aroused before he enters. Expressing your delight in your growing sensitivity and arousal is the best way to communicate with him. If he hears, "Oh, oh, my gosh! Oh, that is so sensitive!" he will slow down, but stay aroused and excited. If you say, "I need you to slow down," especially in a nonerotic voice, he may feel he is being dictated to or worry that he is not pleasing you. His fun and confidence will be affected and he may lose his erection.

G-spot sensitivity, G-spot orgasms, and ejaculating freely will not happen overnight. He'll learn a few things, and you'll give up a few things while you wait for him to catch up. Let him know when he really hits the target. It's helpful to say to your partner, "Oh, oh, oh, pleaaaaase remember that spot!" That gets the message across in an exciting way.

Don't expect him to always remember, but do expect him to catch on after a while.

The great thing about all these positions—and more generally about learning to awaken your G-spot—is the gradualness with which this can occur. Unlike learning to have an orgasm, which often leads people to stuck on one method, variety in how you experience pleasure and orgasm will increase as you slowly incorporate your G-spot awakening into what you already do.

As I said at the beginning of this chapter, the focus on positions will and should drop away over time and will be replaced by a sense of being lost in physical pleasure and emotional connection with your partner. Even ejaculating becomes secondary to that connection. And, unless you are trying to bring a new child into this world or bestow some fortunate fellow with immortality, as in the Quodoushka tradition, I hope ejaculation never becomes the full focus and goal, either.

~ The State of Your Relationship Can ~ Affect Your Ability to Ejaculate

The state of your relationship, and your inner, sexual vitality, will both have the greatest influence on whether you ejaculate. All phases of the life cycle affect desire. A hot affair may bring gushes and gushes of ejaculate; a new romance may make it recede for a time. Ejaculation and emotional G-spot orgasms will ebb and flow with the ebb and flow of a long-term, stable love relationship. And if things aren't going well in your relationship, you could see your desire or ability to ejaculate disappear during that time. The same is true for stressful periods in your life that are not directly caused by the relationship.

But even the bad times can be emoted between partners. Humans need connection as much then as when times are good. Even if the relationship is fragile or ending, if you are still having sex, use your G-spot sensitivity to feel these emotions, too. You don't have to love him, or to scream in joyous ecstasy. Sex is an expression of our moods—all of them. Use your emotional G-spot orgasm to get in touch with your emotions and let it be an expression of your respectful self-love.

~ *The Worst Places to Ejaculate—and Why* ~

Sleeping bags — You might catch cold. It's highly uncomfortable if the bag is flannel, less so if it's made of polypropylene.

The car — Car seats hold stains and possibly smells. Could attract cats.

Your parents' bed — Mortification!

Airplane lavatory — Think about the lack of towels and space to wipe up the mess—a serious head-banging situation.

Your partner's dress slacks — No need to cause undue embarrassment.

Movie theater — You'd be inconsiderate to the next person who sits on that seat (whether ejaculate has healthful properties or not).

~ *The Best Places to Ejaculate—and Why* ~

Motorcycle seat — Wind dries it off almost immediately; ejaculate cools the pipes and drips onto the concrete.

Pickup-truck bed — Who cares?

Hot tub — Adds healthful essences to the healing heat of the water.

Garden — A great compost for the plants.

Ocean — From whence we came.

Most parts of the human body — Especially male bodies. They love it!

⊚ Mopping Up the Mess ⊚

When you start to ejaculate with your partner, you'll probably both wonder how to deal with the large quantities of ejaculate that you can produce. I once received a letter from a woman who asked me if she was damaging herself by ejaculating up to eight times in one lovemaking session. I have heard from women who talk of needing multiple towels, and then more towels, and the bed is still soaked. A demure hanky would probably be preferable for those of us with romantic tastes, but I'm afraid that a hanky can't usually do the job of blotting up all the ejaculate. On the one hand, I'd like to say, "Now girls, let's have fun. This is not the time to worry about the sheets getting all wet and ruined. Yes, there will be traces of stains at times, probably during certain parts of your menstrual cycle." But on the other hand, there's no denying that ejaculate does make a mess. The following are some ideas about how to deal with it:

> *Use towels and blankets.* Usually one thick towel will suffice. I know one woman who had her aqua towel monogrammed with a big "G" and a waterfall. My favorite is a dark-green-and-black-patterned fleece blanket which I fold in half. It covers a large area, is cozy and stays put, and absorbs all the moisture but doesn't soak through quickly.

> *Protect your mattress.* The best and most comfortable way to protect your mattress is to invest in a rubber sheet lined with flannel on one side. Such sheets often are put on a baby's crib. I recommend putting a towel or two over the rubber sheet, as the flannel won't soak up much liquid. If the rubber does not breathe enough for you, an extra-thick mattress pad usually does the trick, if you use a towel under you as well.

> *Invest in Protective Liners.* A professional alternative to towels, blankets, and rubber-backed sheets has recently been created by Karen Fowler, an entrepreneur and mother of two, who hopes to remove a frequent obstacle women face when learning to "let go" into ejaculation—the fear of making a mess. Her Sheet Savers are a wonderful solution for dealing with gooshy sex. The absorbent, waterproof liners are an attractive and affordable way to protect your bed, floors, and carpets. The washable liners (called Luv Liners) come in floral, leopard, or plaid patterns ($22), and the disposable Luv Liners come in peach or beige ($6–$13 per pack). For contact information, please see the Resources section at the back of the book.

> *Aim for your lover.* I get rid of most of my fluid on my boyfriend. He doesn't mind! That makes it fun for me. Since I can ejaculate only when I push out whatever is in my vagina—these days, that's usually his cock—and because my hips usually rise up when I orgasm, the wide berth of his

chest and face and thighs are usually direct targets. Still, if we don't use a towel, the bed usually gets a number of large wet spots on it.

Gulp it down. With oral sex, your partner is often right on the spigot, so to speak. Depending on how much you thrash around when you orgasm, how agile your honey is at catching fluid with his or her lips, and whether drinking your ejaculate is appealing, swallowing could be the tidiest option available.

Have sex in the shower or outdoors. These are wonderful places to have sex anyway, and when you're ejaculating, they are tailor-made to free you from worrying about the mess.

Use an ejaculation bowl. Primarily for ritual use, ejaculation bowls are a wonderful way to collect your ejaculate and study it. As we saw in Chapter 2, many cultures considered the ejaculate to have rejuvenating properties. You can sprinkle it on the garden, use it as a facial treatment, or even drink it. This is not for everyone, but if you like the idea, go for it. I have handmade ejaculation bowls (limited edition) available on my website. (See the Resources section at the back of this book.)

Choose not to ejaculate. Once your waters are truly untapped, it may be unappealing or uncomfortable to not ejaculate. But you can withhold your ejaculate if you are in a "tight spot" where lots of liquid would cause problems. See the sidebar on page 125 for some of the worst, and best, places to ejaculate.

The next chapter will provide more information about ejaculating with a partner and will offer men some tips to help them help you. Remember, always refer back to the times you spent alone awakening your G-spot and learning to ejaculate when you run into obstacles ejaculating in your partnership. Or keep using your time alone as a maintenance tool. The more you experiment, alone and with your partner, the more you'll find you can access and express your ejaculation abilities with comfort and ease.

CHAPTER SEVEN

Men's Role in Female Ejaculation

Jeff was sure his partner was ready to ejaculate. As for him, he was more than ready. He had experienced female ejaculation years ago, and had secretly wished ever since that he could find a woman who would make this happen for him again. Now it seemed his love was about to satisfy this longheld desire.

When his partner, Teresa, said she wanted to learn how to ejaculate (quite out of the blue, it seemed to him), his heart started to pound. He wanted to take off her panties and try right then and there, but held back because he wasn't quite sure what he needed to do for her.

One day soon after her exciting remark, they were making love, and she told him how juicy his caresses had been making her feel lately. She said all he needed to do was go a little slower, and put his finger just inside her vagina during oral sex and rub it slowly. He did this, listening intently to her reactions to this G-spot stimulation. He was so excited by her excitement and by feeling her G-spot growing on his finger, he could barely keep from coming when she asked him to enter her with his penis.

Fighting to control his own orgasm, he could feel her muscles contract forcefully when she had hers. When she pushed him out and ejaculated all over his arms and chest, he felt thrilled!

Jeff was overtaken with desire for her and re-entered her passionately. He came hard and fast with slippery wetness all around, while she

seemed to crave every thrust of his penis. His dreams of finding a woman who would ejaculate for him had come true, and he couldn't stop smiling afterward.

Most men like female ejaculation. Many guys who haven't experienced it might be noncommittal, confused, or even scared off at first when ladies who do ejaculate tell them about it. But once men experience that surprise gush of liquid, they're excited to help it happen again. This chapter will introduce female ejaculation to men who have not had a chance to see what all the excitement is about, and provide information to all men who wish to help with their partners' efforts to ejaculate. Lesbians whose partners ejaculate can learn from this chapter, too.

In this chapter, women will hear from men and women about their experiences with and attitudes toward female ejaculation, and men will hear from women about what they need in order to ejaculate comfortably and with abandon. Women: Point out this chapter to your guy if he is interested in helping you to ejaculate. If he wants even more information, the chapter will direct him to other sections in the book where he can find it. Men: Give this book to your partner if you are excited about female ejaculation and would like to see if she is interested in the subject.

☉ Men Who Love Female Ejaculation and Why ☉

From Paul, a biology student:

> I get off on a woman who gushes on me. And at times, the taste of it
> isn't bad at all.

From Mikaya, lesbian author:

> The first time I experienced a woman ejaculating, I was hit in the chest
> by a stream of fluid as I sat between my lover's legs with my fingers
> inside her. I'd never heard of ejaculation, but I thought it was the
> hottest thing that had happened to me in a long time, and I didn't care
> whether it was pee or not. I pretty soon realized it wasn't, since it
> neither looked nor smelled like pee. I wanted to repeat it right away,
> and I'm happy to say I did get to repeat it a number of times.

From John Setchell, maker of an award-winning documentary in England on female ejaculation:

> My partner and I were "at it" in a hotel room one afternoon—we had been looking forward to it all day and hadn't even paused to take the duvet off the bed! She had several intense but "dry" orgasms sitting on top of me and then came and ejaculated a huge amount that flowed for several seconds and soaked me, the duvet, the bottom sheet, and the undersheet, right down to the mattress. If we had poured a glass of water onto the bed, it wouldn't have done all that!

From an anonymous person responding to my website:

> I love the gush!

From Russell, a Canadian computer specialist:

> What I enjoy most about the experience is that my partner is really letting go, that trust and intimacy exist between us to such an extent that there is no holding back, that it is safe to surrender to pleasure, without inhibition.

One young man from France e-mailed that he regards his own ejaculation as a sign of love for his partner, and sees female ejaculation the same way:

> It's a sign that she loves you without having to say anything. In my experience, I love to give pleasure with caresses and licking my partner. If I get my partner to ejaculate, my pleasure is immense.

Jack, a friend who lives in Oregon, echoes the same sentiments about female ejaculation communicating love:

> Although female ejaculation may not be for everyone, when it happens, I always feel like it is a wonderful and very sexy gift, and it's really a turn-on! To me, the very deepest part of her is saying "Yes!!" to the quality of our connection in that moment, and it sends our lovemaking into a more blissful and much deeper intimacy.

From an anonymous response to my website:

I think for most men, female ejaculation is an oddity. The first time I experienced this phenomenon, I was amazed and incredibly excited over the response experienced by the woman I was with. The idea of something "gushing" from a woman's pussy [actually the urethra] other than urine or the typical lubrication for penetration was thrilling. What is truly awesome is the distance that a woman can expel this fluid and the intensity with which she does this. Obviously, female ejaculation is more intense than the "usual" orgasm that a woman has.

From a Vietnam veteran :

It's sensual, cool. Especially when she gets all wild and carried away. It lets me know my honey feels real good.

From Frank, a filmmaker:

I heard this story about a woman who gushed on a new lover, and he was shocked and lost his erection. They went their separate ways, and she thought she would not hear from him again. However, he phoned her a few days later, saying that he had done some research on the Internet about what had happened and now understood about FE. He found it exciting but had to "get his head around it" and asked when could he please see her again!

From Josh, a wilderness guide:

My only exposure to female ejaculation was when I was quite young— early twenties—and not very aware. I was with a woman who, on our second or third date, got naked and masturbated—under the auspices of doing it for me, but really it was for her. I was totally unprepared for her ejaculation, and it surprised—and soaked—me. While it was apparently common for her, she hadn't communicated what to expect and I had no idea if she was urinating or what was going on. I lost my erection and felt confused and insecure. Since I didn't "rise to the occasion" (in more ways than one, so to speak), that was the last I heard from her. Ahh, the insecurities of my youth!

From Don, a retired engineer, now a Peruvian whistle bowl maker:

My first experience was only recently. I assisted my new love in experiencing yet another orgasm without being inside her. I noticed that immediately after her orgasmic cresting, a flood of warm fluid washed across my fingers. I immediately experienced a warm sensual rush of feeling. It was, in a manner I can't express in words, "charged" with warm, sensual, feminine energy. There was no question in my mind that it wasn't urine, because of its energy and viscosity. It was clearly *not* urine and was welcomed by me and fulfilling on a very deep and instinctive level.

From Michael, an avid golfer and metal manufacturer:

What I like is the feeling of my partner reaching a level of pleasure, a climax to her pleasure, that manifests itself in this explosive release of her juices from within her body. The feeling of that explosion, the hot liquid which she gives to me, which feels so exquisite on the erogenous parts of my body, gets me so orgasmic that there can be this simultaneous cumming explosion where we are releasing, giving ourselves to each other in a way that may be the ultimate feeling of eros.

From David, a writer:

I was with this woman who filled one of her high-heeled shoes with her ejaculate. We couldn't stop laughing. The shoe was full to the brim, not counting what was all over the carpet!

From Sophia, a bisexual health-care professional:

It's such a turn on; I love getting all wet! It helped to show me how much my girlfriend really enjoyed our lovemaking. I think ejaculation may be more common between two women because there isn't the final goal of penis intercourse. I think we get more creative with fingers and tongues. When you get that spot and she releases her juices all over you—there's just nothing else like it! I wish I could do it, too. Someday I will.

⊚ Women Who Love Men Who Love ⊚ Female Ejaculation and Why

It seems that our lovers, on the whole, have far fewer problems accepting the notion that women ejaculate than we ourselves do, and men are even eager to have the experience in their lives. This open and supportive attitude is great for a woman when she is first learning how to ejaculate, especially if he doesn't pressure her to ejaculate right away. Here are a few more stories from men and women about what support or the lack of it can do to a woman who is trying to ejaculate. They also illustrate women's ability to hold back ejaculation and even to alter their sexual behavior as a result of this rejection.

From Anatolia, an herbalist:

> I love it that my partner is so comfortable with my ejaculating. I wasn't sure how he would react to being sprayed. I mean, who wants a bath every time they make love. But that doesn't seem to bother him, and it's helped me loosen up even more and feel free to enjoy myself.

Mary, contributor to the online G-spot chat group:

> A woman I know with a high sex drive had ejaculated regularly, from her first orgasm in her early teens. She had received various reactions to this from her lovers. She married a guy who "tolerated," but was unenthusiastic about, female ejaculation, and over a period of time she came to believe FEing was wrong, and her sex drive diminished. Eventually it caused the end of her marriage. Now she is with a guy who understands and enjoys FE, and her sexual pleasure and energy have returned.

Bill, writing to the G-spot chat group:

> My girlfriend told me she had [once] been on a few dates with a man, and they had gone away for the weekend to have sex together for the first time. She liked him, was very excited, orgasmed strongly, and ejaculated on him. She had experienced FE before but didn't intend to

do it this time, but she just couldn't help herself. He was appalled, insisted that they both get dressed and pack, and drove her back to the rail station! She never heard from him or saw him again.

A friend, Connie, an architect, writes:

I ejaculated freely with my partner of six years without [any] thought of it being a problem. Toward the end of the relationship, I sensed it was turning him off. Immediately, I noticed I ejaculated far less. Since I was aware I could control my ejaculate, I began to not ejaculate at all at times. After the relationship ended, I didn't ejaculate for four years. I guess I felt rejected and just didn't want to. For a while I thought I couldn't ejaculate anymore, but I came to realize I just felt undesirable after our parting.

Margie, an English woman I chatted with over the Internet about female ejaculation, describes her desire to burst all over her partner with abandon:

Secretly inside me, I wish I could blow all over again and again and feel completely free, like it is so normal.

A woman writes to the G-spot chat group:

I was making love with a friend of mine and this [ejaculation] happened to me. He quickly got up and changed the sheets. I was humiliated and really hurt. I told him this was an ejaculation, but he insisted I had urinated on the bed.

A friend of mine, Angie, had a reassuring experience when she first ejaculated with her husband years ago:

I had an awesome orgasm, and suddenly I felt this rush out of me and this stuff was spraying out of my body. I thought I'd peed, but thought, "Well, maybe I peed because the orgasm was so intense." The bed was soaking wet; it was a mess. It surprised him too, but we continued to have sex. Afterwards, I told him, "I peed in the bed." He said, "I don't think you peed in the bed, because it doesn't smell. It's your smell, Angie. Remember I always say I could find you anywhere;

I could find you in a crowded room?" I asked him if I smelled that bad.
He laughed and said, "No, it's just you, your smell." I thought, "Wow!
I'd been carrying that stuff around for a long time!" Neither one of us
knew then about the G-spot or ejaculation or anything.

◉ Helping a Woman to Ejaculate Successfully ◉

When your partner first tells you about her interest in female ejaculation,
it is wise to take a back seat, keep an open mind, and see what transpires.
Let her get used to the idea, and encourage her to experiment and develop
her abilities on her own for a while.

I recommend that women learn how to ejaculate on their own at first,
because the solo exercises offered in Chapters 4, 5, and 6 offer detailed
information on how to find the G-spot, how to stimulate it, and how to
build and expel ejaculate fluid. Once female ejaculation is achieved in this
solo manner, a woman will have more success ejaculating with a partner.
But if she insists that you get involved earlier in her explorations, the
following are some things you can do:

- Become familiar with G-spot anatomy and how to stimulate her
  G-spot. (Consult the sections in Chapter 4 on finding and stimulating the G-spot (pages 81–85), and see "Surefire Techniques,"
  later in this chapter.)

- Encourage her to tell you what she likes, especially if she doesn't
  usually speak up.

- Have a sense of humor and don't be goal-oriented; most
  women like ejaculation and want to ejaculate, but for them it's
  less a goal than part of the overall experience of making love.

All of the attempts you make, even if they don't result in ejaculation, move
both of you farther along the learning curve and increase the likelihood of
eventual success.

Women like to include their partners in activities, and sexuality is no
exception. But from a woman's perspective, men can be too enthusiastic and
rush into "getting the job done." Nothing prevents ejaculation more

effectively than pressure to ejaculate! Most women need time to talk about female ejaculation, to explore its twists and turns, before they actually attempt it. As I've said throughout this book, they will have the best chances of success if their first explorations are made solo. So, for example, if she expresses interest in ejaculating, say something like, "Oh, have you ever done that before?" or "Where did you hear about that?" This may seem evasive to you, but such questions can help her figure out exactly what she wants to do.

If she complains about not being able to ejaculate, or if she's wishing she could, say something like, "Oh, that sounds interesting" or "Did you hear or read something about that?" Keep asking questions for a while. When she answers, the best response is to reflect back to her what she just said. For example, if she says, "I've been hearing about it from a friend," respond by saying, "So you've got some new information. What did she tell you?"

Drawing her out further is wise, even if what she's said seems plain enough to you, because she's giving you a signal to talk, rather than a signal to act. So take time to discuss female ejaculation before you jump in and try to help out with something that she may not yet be ready to attempt. This can help you to avoid a frustrating first experience in which you both end up feeling like you've failed.

The following section sums up a lot of the information from the rest of this book. It also might be a good idea to read Chapter 4, which has more details about how a woman assesses her readiness to ejaculate and how she can learn and practice ejaculating on her own.

Before you begin trying to help her ejaculate, check the following three things:

Strength of her PC muscles. An essential point: Your partner can't ejaculate if her vaginal (PC) muscles are weak. Some guys think that a woman with a loose vagina has, as one man told me, "screwed around too much," but that is not the case. A loose vagina just indicates that her PC muscles are weak from lack of exercise. Trying to get her to ejaculate will be a frustrating experience until her PC muscles are tightened and strengthened. If her vagina feels loose during intercourse, that's a sure sign that she needs to do PC exercises—have a look at Chapter 5, where these exercises are explained. Encourage her to do them, and to practice them on your love tool, too! Having stronger PC muscles not only feels great for both of you, it encourages all around vaginal health. When you both feel that her vagina is tighter when you have sex, that is a signal that she is ready, muscle-wise at least, to attempt to ejaculate.

~ *Don't Bruise the Grapes* ~

A woman who can firmly clamp down on your penis is nice, as you know, but feeling the firmness of a full and bursting G-spot against your penis is even better! Consider the G-spot a small bunch of tiny, very full and juicy grapes. But don't bruise the grapes! Make them burst instead! Your penis is their sunshine, and when the grapes are nourished, they become fully ripened orbs containing juices that will burst all over you!

Her attitude toward ejaculate. Letting go is the aspect of female ejaculation that is most difficult for most women to master. If she is afraid she is going to urinate on you and that you will be upset, she will have a hard time ejaculating. Reassure her more than once: "It probably won't be urine, and if it is, I don't care."

Deep-seated sexual issues. Awakening the G-spot is an important step in a woman's sexual life, and it can bring up all kinds of emotional issues. If a woman shuts down abruptly once she begins learning to ejaculate, give her some time away from ejaculating for a while. Reassure her by saying, "It's okay if you don't ejaculate." If she continues to distance you sexually, check out Chapter 8—there may be some deeper issues involved.

Once you feel that she may be ready to attempt ejaculation, ask her if she wants your help. If she says yes, check again, asking in a caring tone: "Are you sure?" This is not a put-down; it's just a confirmation for both of you. If you are greeted with another affirmative, the next section will help you to discover where her G-spot is and how to help her ejaculate.

☉ **Surefire Techniques** ☉

Guys are usually up for sexually pleasing their honeys, and most men approach female ejaculation for the first time with an open mind. But if you are called upon to actually help a woman ejaculate, you might feel uncomfortable because you aren't sure what to do or you don't understand how female ejaculation works. So, guys, I've tried to make this as simple and direct as possible to help you out here. For more lengthy information, take a look at Chapter 2, which discusses women's anatomy in detail. In the meantime, meet the G-Man, a cartoon character on the hunt for the G-spot, in *The Adventures of G-Man and the Gushing Caves.*

FIND THE G-SPOT

These are the adventures of a character known as the G-Man, friend of the ladies and a great explorer. He's just put on a rain slicker and galoshes, and set off to investigate rumors of gushing caves.

He finds a cave, walks up to it, and takes a step inside. The cave is shaped like a long tunnel. Through the darkness, he can faintly see a back wall. He looks up and sees a flattened-out rocket strapped to the cave's ceiling. Its nose cone is butted up to the entrance to the cave, and its body extends over a third or more of the cave's ceiling. He can see its tail. He walks over to the tail and pushes on its end. The rocket starts to rev up.

The rocket's underbelly is interesting: It's covered in miniature ripples like corrugated sheet metal but the surface feels slick and warm. He pushes on it and notices that it gives like a firm sponge. All kinds of torque and acceleration buttons are set into the nose cone, belly, and tail. He pushes these buttons to find out what they will do, and the rocket revs up and down. After a while, he observes that pushing these buttons also makes the rocket's belly and nose grow bigger and swell, and now he has to crouch down a little.

He finds a few buttons that rev up the rocket to high speed. The rocket's surface gets hot and so slick that it starts to drip, and he starts to sweat. He notices that the rocket is starting to tilt. Looking closer, he sees it's not really tilting but changing its shape. The tail flattens out into the roof of the cave, and the nose swells downward, almost filling the cave entrance—getting out will be a tight squeeze. The rocket looks like it's positioning itself for launch. The nose cone and belly are loaded up, and the whole thing feels like it's about to take off and thunder out of the cave.

He sets all the buttons on max rev to see if the rocket will launch. He's not quite sure what is going to happen. The cave is starting to rumble and shake. He decides that he had better get out. The entrance is tight but it's slippery as heck, so he slides and tumbles out. Suddenly, it seems a dam just broke loose behind him. He's swept up and jostled around, pelted relentlessly with a pounding shower.

Just as suddenly as they started, things calm down. He looks around. The rocket's still on the roof of the cave, but now water is dripping out of the hole in the center of the rocket's nose. The rocket is powering down. It flattens again, shudders, and turns off. The G-Man stands there dripping, and he grins because, while that was a close call, he completed his mission and explored the gushing cave.

STIMULATE THE G-SPOT

Now that you know where the G-spot is, here is a yellow road sign to guide you when you begin to stimulate her G-spot:

WARNING!

SENSITIVE AREA!

PROCEED SLOWLY!

These first few techniques are not all that erotically thrilling for her or you, but they will help you understand where her pleasure points are, and help her to become aware of the sensitivity of her G-spot. They are great techniques to use when you first begin to stimulate her G-spot, and they require some preliminary stimulation, for example, using oral sex. If oral sex is not a part of your foreplay, stimulate her clitoris (lightly) with your fingers. If rapid vaginal stimulation with your fingers is your usual method, try lightly teasing her vulva and clitoris with your fingers instead, then begin.

~ All Women Have a G-Spot ~

Don't be fooled into thinking she doesn't have a G-spot, even if you try to stimulate it a few times and she doesn't feel anything. Every woman has one! If your partner says she cannot feel anything, it's best to stop trying and ask her to read and practice Chapters 4 and 5. (Chapter 4 is also a good chapter for you if you want further details on stimulation techniques.)

Come Here Honey. This method is a basic way to stimulate her G-spot. After you have aroused her with some slow, teasing oral sex or foreplay, slowly slip your finger into her wet and ready vagina. Slide carefully along the upper wall (versus the bottom) of the vagina until you feel the curl of the G-spot's tail described in the G-Man story. Once you find the tail, push firmly and massage it.

A variation on this massage method is a "come hither" approach, described by Robin, a friend of mine:

> I have always been aware of my G-spot, and my husband knows instinctively when to start stimulating it—once I'm truly wet! Insert your middle finger, palm up, and use a "come here" motion to rub the top wall of her vagina. She will soon become aware of the most blissful sensations!

Play Me Baby. Repeat the above method, but press firmly all around the G-spot in fractional movements, stopping to ask her what she feels as you hold your finger still in one spot. If she feels nothing, massage this area on the G-spot slowly and firmly. Note her reaction and move on to the next area. I like this description of the Play Me Baby method by Michael, a musician:

> I can feel her respond as I alter the way I touch her—the intensity, and where exactly I touch her, is like playing an instrument in a duo and listening, being sensitive to the dynamics and all the nuances being put forth by the person you're playing with.

Love in the Gutter. Run your finger like a window washer across the body of the G-spot. While you are doing it, ask her how it feels. Your goal is to notice how the G-spot's body dips down on each side, creating a gutter between the body and the vaginal wall. Insert two fingers, one on each side, and rub the gutters, moving in and out slowly, a couple of times. Ask her what she feels. (You can find a fuller description of this method in the Chapter 4 section, "Find Your G-Spot.")

~ *If She Says She Doesn't Feel Anything* ~

If your partner has never found her G-spot or ejaculated, she may be completely unaware of its sensitivity. Believe me, if you are rubbing the upper vaginal wall as described in this section, you are rubbing her G-spot, even if she doesn't feel anything.

If your partner cannot feel G-spot sensations, assess the situation with this simple test. Using your fingers during foreplay, get a sense of the size of her prostate gland (G-spot) by feeling the upper vaginal wall, from the vaginal opening to where the bulge of the G-spot stops,. Measure once when she is not aroused and a second time when she is. See if you can detect any increase in the size of her prostate/G-spot—and ask her what she feels, too! If you notice the G-spot is larger with arousal, no worries! From here, it will be a matter of awakening the G-spot's sensitivity. Continue using all the methods described in this chapter to slowly but surely awaken her spot.

If you cannot feel any increase in size, it is likely she will not ejaculate any time soon. There are a few possible reasons for this: 1) the stimulation is incorrect, or too brief, 2) she is not really aroused, 3) she is one of the 10 percent of women who have a very small G-spot or a G-spot located toward the back of the vagina's ceiling, or 4) she has not yet awakened to the natural sensitivity of her G-spot. Continue all methods described in this chapter in order to slowly but surely awaken her spot and/or encourage her to read and practice the solo explorations described in Chapter 4.

With time, it may be possible to feel "nodules" in the body of the G-spot. A psychologist wrote to me and described what he feels as his partner's G-spot becomes aroused:

> I can feel these little "peas" through the vaginal roof, almost like a bunch of tiny water balloons that are at first empty, then fill up, and then deflate again after she ejaculates.

EXPELL THE EJACULATE MANUALLY

Once you have found her G-spot, things get a little more exciting. This next method is an advanced technique in which you will manually help her ejaculate. Once you are knowledgeable about and adept at stimulating her G-spot, *and* you notice it becoming swollen and sensitive, you can "milk the pod" to achieve ejaculation. Your likelihood of success increases dramatically if you arouse her using more G-spot than clitoral stimulation.

> *Milk the pod*—It may be possible to get your partner to ejaculate the first time, without an orgasm, by manually stimulating the prostate gland and "milking out" the ejaculate. Use the three methods described above to stimulate the G-spot, and then add some penetration stimulation (described below in the "Lovehandle Massage" and "Heads Up" sections). When her G-spot has enlarged in size and she is aroused, use your fingers and apply a "milking" motion from the tail of the G-spot down along its body. Alternate the milking motion with a gentle but firm "squeezing and rolling," pressing from the gutters.

Cautionary note: This level of stimulation is not recommended if your partner doesn't know what you are doing, and certainly not if she has reservations about ejaculating. She has to help you by physically pushing and/or mentally allowing the ejaculate to flow. Without this, the technique is likely to fail, causing discomfort and possibly bladder infections, because it leaves her with a lot of built-up fluid. Think blue balls!

~ *How Much Ejaculate You Can Expect* ~

Here is what a male friend told me about how much ejaculate may be awaiting you in the treasure of her G-spot, although smaller amounts are more likely at first and are completely normal:

> My love is able to ejaculate from several teaspoons to as much as a half a cup of liquid. The principal way that this occurs is with digital stimulation of the G-spot, or with our usual type of penetrative sex. My love has been able to ejaculate multiple times within a short period of time, probably two to four times in a minute if she is properly stimulated and in the mood.

Sound fun?

G-SPOT STIMULATION AND EJACULATION DURING LOVEMAKING

Use your lovehandle—your cock—to try the following G-spot-awakening maneuvers. These techniques will help you become more aware of how your penis is stimulating her G-spot to create ejaculate.

Lovehandle Massage. Use the lip on the head of your penis and massage the tail end of her G-spot. Go very slowly at first, hardly moving, until you both can feel the G-spot. Slowly try to roll, rub, and massage the tail of the G-spot with your penis as you did with your fingers, in and out, side to side, and all around, in fractional movements. You can increase the speed after a few sessions, but if you go too fast she may lose the sensation. If she does, simply slow back down and proceed.

Heads Up. Use the head of your penis to rub the body of her G-spot. Then try to locate the most sensitive area. For some women, this area may be barely inside the vaginal entrance. If so, gently and slowly pull out and push in. It's very exciting to use the rim of your penis to stimulate this area. Other women may like it a little farther inside the vagina, or outside the vagina and near, or on, the urethral opening. If your partner tenses up, remind her to relax and take a deep breath. Notice the difference in her response when her vagina is relaxed and when it is tense.

As my friend Elaine confided to me in a delicious session of girl talk:

> I love when he goes slow and I can relax. It is like sensations directly
> from his penis I never felt before. It gets so intense I want to scream
> and bite! I've learned to breath and relax into this intense pleasure,
> and it builds to such a point in me that my orgasm got so intense a
> few times I literally saw stars. After that kind of physical release, which
> always seems to have a lot of ejaculate, he's my shining star, for sure!

Once things have moved on to the point where both of you are experiencing the pleasure of a full and juicy G-spot, you will be able to enjoy the full range and intensity of exciting sexual connection! Four great sexual positions are described in the "The Best Sexual Positions for Ejaculating" section in Chapter 6. Read those now to get more ideas for having fun with the G-spot and success with ejaculation during lovemaking. Then come back and read the following descriptions of two couples enjoying female ejaculation—to keep you motivated for when your honey's G-spot goes full throttle:

John Setchell remembers his first time:

> The first time I experienced FE we were doing 69, with my partner
> above me. I had several fingers inside her and was stimulating her
> G-spot by pressing down toward my face when suddenly she gushed
> all over my face and chest. It was thrilling! Next evening, we spent
> some time paying attention to how it had occurred, and we quickly
> learned what we needed to do to make it happen regularly.

Nan, a butch videographer, likes to have it this way:

> Have her on top, on her knees over you, with her titties in your face
> and your dick or fingers in her pussy. This way it's easy to massage
> her G-spot, and when she comes, her hot fluid runs over your belly
> and chest. Super-intimate; that's why I like it—face-to-face sharing of
> that G-spot moment.

All these methods may not produce amazing results the first time you try them. If a huge fountain of ejaculate does occur, consider yourself fortunate. It might take many tries over a considerable period of time to get a woman to ejaculate even a small amount, because you are helping to awaken an area which in many women has shrunk or shut down from nonuse, or that has been numbed out from too much intensive thrusting.

The most successful approach, therefore, is to incorporate these methods into your lovemaking, making progress bit by bit, as both of you explore. This gradual process of awakening the G-spot to create ejaculation is physically pleasurable, and each time it will feel like something new has happened sexually between the two of you. Enjoy the process!

◎ Male Multiple Orgasms Assist ◎ Female Ejaculation

The kind of stimulation necessary to awaken her G-spot and build ejaculate fluid requires slowing down and is contrary to the masculine desire to come with urgency, fire, and passion. However, there are major benefits to slowing down: She'll open up more and be more satisfied, and you get to stay hard longer and have multiple orgasms. Once you taste the pleasures that can arise from adopting a slower approach to lovemaking, you may find that using a slow fire with increased intensity becomes preferable to your tried-and-true type of release.

The best way to retain the fire and relax into a slower buildup of pleasure that lasts for an extended period of time is to become multi-orgasmic. Through this highly pleasurable practice, a man learns to separate his ejaculation response from his orgasms. Learning to have these nonejaculatory multi-orgasms is not any more difficult for men than learning to combine ejaculation *with* their orgasms is for women.

In their book, *The Art of Conscious Loving,* Tantric pioneers and workshop leaders Charles and Caroline Muir see many benefits to men in learning ejaculation awareness. One benefit is that "a man who exercises this kind of control often seems to give the woman freedom to finally lose control of herself."

What's more, the physical, emotional, and mental letdown that most men experience after sex is absent when men have an orgasm without ejaculating, because ejaculating is what drains men of their energy. Without ejaculation, most men find that their energy level stays high after sex. This is good news for women, too, who are often left frustrated without an orgasm because the man came too soon, and saddened by his sudden withdrawal after his orgasm.

Victor Gold, who appeared in my video *Tantric Journey to Female Orgasm*, has been practicing ejaculation control for more than twenty years. Now fifty-five years old, he explains his views on increased vitality through ejaculation control:

> When I do ejaculate, which is rare, I am aware of having tremendous loss of energy. Some men can ejaculate more than others and still retain their vitality. I've done a lot of research on this aspect of ejaculation control. Basically, frequency of ejaculation would best be determined by the age, health, fitness level, and stress level of the individual. So, older, more unhealthy men have to ejaculate less, and younger, more healthy men can ejaculate more.

For men and women who have read this far through this book, it will be easy enough to understand how it is entirely possible to have an orgasm and not ejaculate. The task for both men and women is to become aware of the ejaculate urges; women must learn that they do arise and how to open further to them, and men must learn when the ejaculate is about to rise up and how to quell it.

The technique that allows men to separate orgasm from ejaculation is easy enough to learn, but learning to control the urge is, as I'm sure I don't have to tell you, more difficult. One man I talked with put the whole process of learning how to do this very simply: "Nonejaculation at orgasm can be learned (I can do it) by training the PC muscles in the prostate area not to spasm at orgasm." This is exactly what women have unconsciously learned to do in order not to ejaculate.

There are a few techniques you can learn to keep yourself from ejaculating—and still have an orgasm:

🌀 Just as you become aware you are about to ejaculate, stop all movement and ask her to stop as well. Push your finger firmly against

the place between your anus and scrotum called the "perineum."
Wait until the urge subsides, and then continue on.

🖎 You can also grab your penis tightly around its rim under the
head, or you can encircle your balls with your hand and pull down.
Once you get used to controlling the urge to ejaculate, you'll be
able to dispense with these methods and do it with breathing.

A sexy audiotape called *Be the Man of Her Fantasies!* by Maryse Cote
(also known as the Canadian vixen Ishtara) is guaranteed to make your
first exposure to male ejaculation control erotic! (Good luck controlling
it with her incredible voice and attitude at the helm. However, I highly
recommend a visit with her!) Excellent books on the ancient belief that
withholding ejaculation increases men's vitality, as well as further
details on how to accomplish ejaculation control, are Mantak Chia's
Taoist Secrets of Love: Cultivating Male Sexual Energy and *The Multi-
Orgasmic Man*. (See the Resources section at the back of this book for
more information on male ejaculation control guides.)

Until very recently, it used to be that male ejaculation control
methods such as these were the only choices available for men who
wanted to slow down in order to assist a partner in her G-spot orgasm
or to enter into higher states of sexual energy exchange. But male ejaculation control is modeled on an outmoded stereotype of men needing
to "control" themselves. In truth, male ejaculation control too often
feels more like torture than pleasure to most men, and it increases
performance pressures rather than alleviating them. These drawbacks to
male ejaculation control methods can stifle the very effects they are
meant to enhance: losing oneself in connection and erotic pleasure. Too
often male ejaculation control can feel more like distancing oneself
further from the sex act in order to slow down enough to satisfy one's
female partner.

Jack Johnston, M.A., advocates male multiple orgasms over ejaculation control. The technique he teaches does not require any squeeze or
withhold method and eliminates the sensation of having to hold back
the ejaculate energy. Instead it concentrates on opening up to more

pleasure, which can cascade into having more than one orgasm. I highly recommend his excellent audio CD, *Male Multiple Orgasm,* as an introduction to this new world of pleasure for men. He offers on-going support on his website www.multiples.com via weekly internet chats and through audio testimonials and Q &A from other men who are learning to bypass the frustrating ejaculation control method and just have multiple orgasms. He is also listed in the back of the book in the Resource section under the section, "For Men: More Pleasure, Less Control."

Fiery passion will still occur with male multiple orgasms, but it will have different flavor and timing. As your partner gains greater sensitivity in her G-spot over perhaps many years of lovemaking, her G-spot may feel uncomfortable and sensitive before she is aroused. Imagine having your prostate touched without erotic arousal; it's not very appealing. A woman will flinch in the same manner to cold, rough touch on her unaroused, yet awakened (sensitized) prostate. To rush into sex at this point causes her G-spot to shut down and numb out— like the clitoris does if it is overstimulated. However, once a woman with a sensitized prostate (G-spot) is aroused and truly ready for intercourse, she'll welcome deep and passionate thrusting.

So, thrusting will not be a thing of the past, but its timing will be different. Allow a woman extra time to juice up her G-spot and she will open her heart to you and be much more satisfied with her sexual interactions than she's ever been before. In addition, men who become multi-orgasmic can enter into a realm of greater intimacy that comes with mixing their deepest emotions with erotic passion. This is the first step toward experiencing what the ancients called "being blessed with Immortality."

◌ Entering the Temple of Love ◌

G-spot stimulation and orgasms are emotional by nature. Emotions have not, traditionally, been men's preferred territory, but if you want to help a woman ejaculate, it's best to understand how emotions are connected to a G-spot orgasm. A woman who wrote to me after seeing my video had this to say about emotions and the deeply satiating experience of her G-spot orgasms:

> I try to [protect] a man's ego and his erection, as we women have
> been taught, by being nice. [If I don't get] enough time to get aroused
> and orgasm deeply and ejaculate, I'll slough it off. But the fact is I am
> much happier when I have an orgasm. It's like I can move along.
> Otherwise, things feel stuck, not just orgasmically but emotionally and
> mentally. I get resentment that is hard to let go of. It is freeing to have
> a G-spot orgasm, emote, and ejaculate, and I notice I'm happier.

Men and women are often turned on by different things. The basic difference is best described by Charles and Caroline Muir in their book, *Tantra: The Art of Conscious Loving*. They explain that women, in general, interpret "sexual intimacy" as relating more to the heart or soul than to intercourse, but "when true sexual intimacy for women does occur, sexual passion is its by-product." On the other hand, what typically arouses men, in general, is the thought of intercourse. If the stimulus that most turns on a woman is missing, she remains unsatisfied at a primal level, and loses interest in sex.

Karan is a young friend who wrote to me explaining why she isn't interested in sex or men lately. What she has to say is strikingly illustrative of the Muir's explanation of how women create sexual arousal from a "heart" or soul connection, and how they yearn for emotional and energetic connection:

> Arousal. Getting off...it means nothing to me anymore. What I want is
> intellectual intercourse. Spiritual arousal. Someone who really ignites a
> passion in me, makes the nerves shake....

Emotional safety is a big factor in helping women let go in order to ejaculate. Safety means feeling free to let all her emotions out, to be her real self and be acknowledged with a mutual response, without it being interrupted by the male's ejaculation long before she is ready. This letter from Ana, another young woman who took my workshop, to her lover, reveals more about the connection between feeling emotionally safe enough to reveal her true self and a woman's G-spot orgasm:

My G-spot is right there, at the opening, loaded with sensation. Intense, nasty, loving. Dying to be caressed and opened up, to know that I am safe with you and that you understand and allow my emotions to come forth. You always want to drive me wild and ecstatic with your hardness—the way you found my G-spot and purposely rubbed it with your cock—and I surrender into the sensations from your touch of love; it feels so exquisite to me. I have felt that "G-spot sensation" before, briefly, but never connected it to my G-spot or to love, so its sensation never grew. Now, I see it grows with awareness, and now that the awareness is upon me, I want this kind of sexual connection more and more.

A word of warning about unleashing female desire through G-spot stimulation and orgasm: It is emotional and it is starved. I have spoken to so many women who crave this emotional connection with their partners in sex. Your erotic skill with her G-spot will allow her to express a deep need that has been missing or that has been misdirected for a lot of women into frustration and irritation, due to the different feelings that men and women have about the meaning of intimacy and to the fact that the anatomical trigger for a woman's heart- and soul-based eroticism—the G-spot—has been believed to be "as real as a UFO."

Be prepared for these emotional outpourings and longings. They are a signal to share your heart and to listen to what hers wants to say to you. It may be confusing, but take time to figure out how to handle this. Here is how one experienced G-Man deals with the emotion that G-spot stimulation can create. Raul is an actor and low-impact forester who lives in Northern California and who appeared in my video *Tantric Journey to Female Orgasm: Awaken Your G-Spot*:

I don't jump into sex. I treat sex as a place to break through to. I change my goal to just being in bed, not orgasm. When she gets emotional, I laugh and sing to her.

Saul, an actor, aged sixty-five says:

Once intimate and in a comfortable place together, and she is happy and full of pleasure (which I've done by kissing her slowly and caress-

ing her), I wait until her G-spot is ready and ripe. I just touch it then,
gently, and waves of pleasure go through her body. By that time, it's
intuitive and I don't need to think. I just know what to do. It's like fire-
works then.

The G-spot is literally the heart of women's erotic desire. What to do?
Follow the road sign:

WARNING!

SENSITIVE AREA!

PROCEED SLOWLY!

This temple of love is full of mystery and precious jewels. Be adoring and
playful, talk, listen, and slow down. Soon, the treasure is yours to enjoy.

To enter the temple of love—emotional, connective G-spot lovemaking—you must focus on experiencing the connection. Then, as if by magic,
your erection will take care of itself, and the more attention your lovehandle will end up getting. In other words, the more you slow down, the more
you feel. Learning nonejaculation multi-orgasms will reward a man with a
shower of happiness, radiance, and attention from his partner, as well as the
thrill of her ejaculate on his belly.

This focus on connection with your partner and the erotic pleasure
found in slowing down will also open the door to multiple orgasms for you.
Robert suffered a spinal cord injury in an auto accident and found that
ejaculation caused him a lot of pain. He learned how to control his ejaculation through studying with Jack Johnston, and he has this to say on
Johnston's "Male Multiple Orgasm" audio CD:

It feels like I was meant to be doing this my whole life. It feels
completely natural. Especially because of my injury, ejaculatory orgasm
is really draining for me, but each multiple orgasm actually feels charg-
ing and afterwards I feel awake and aware, erotically charged and
happy all day. I feel more content in general, mostly because it took
away the tension in our relationship that wasn't on the surface, but

was there, because I guess I always felt I had to catch up with women
sexually. I learned to last as long as possible by holding back—while
she had many orgasms—to the point where I couldn't even finish
sometimes. I thought that was the best I could ever do, but now I've
gone *way* past that. These multi-orgasms that give me so much more
pleasure have also helped me control the pain and actually begin to
heal from my injury as well.

Having danced on men's laps, as well as on stage, I know that men,
not just women, yearn for emotional connection and the thrill of embracing in passionate erotic bliss. The sexual entertainment houses and
websites are packed with men looking for that one image or connection
that will fulfil their hunger for mutual sexual excitement and uninhibited
abandon. I have talked to too many men who are also in pain, searching
for something more.

Every caress on a woman's G-spot presents the opportunity for
genuine human connection. If you approach the G-spot and female ejaculation as just another manual technique to perform, and your lovemaking primarily as sport sex, you lose this opportunity to connect. However
deeply you wish to experience sexual intimacy, know that understanding
women's soulful eroticism and its expression, via the G-spot, is one solution to the age-old problem of men and women having a difficult time
satisfying each other emotionally and sexually.

If your partner wishes to inhabit this realm with you but finds she is
running into serious snags, the next chapter explains how you can help
her get over the obstacles that could be holding her back from becoming
your equal, uninhibited partner in sex and in life. This process, like the
ones you've just learned, will help you find the connection you seek from
her, as well.

embracing *the*
FEMININE SPRING

CHAPTER EIGHT

Heal Your G-Spot

◆

A friend of mine, Melinda, is a recently divorced woman in her early fifties with long, sandy hair and a lean body, fit from frequent hikes in the high desert of the Southwest and lots of yoga and meditation. Her new freedom is allowing her to explore her sexuality for the first time in her life. She decided to find her G-spot, and after a few tries, called up her new lover, exclaiming, "I found it!"

She showed him what she had discovered, and asked him to remember exactly where it was. When he felt her G-spot, she experienced a rush of warm love that felt both physical and emotional; it all seemed to be rolled into one big sensation. Then, as if she had decided that were enough for now, she quit experimenting. However, she continued to talk about it for many months, leaving me to wonder what other emotions she might have felt as well.

A few months later, she confided to me that she felt overwhelmed by her longing for this intimate, emotional connection with someone she loved, and also fearful at the possibility of getting it. Her pain was deep and she fought to hold back tears. She said she hadn't connected the exploration of her G-spot with these feelings, but now understood why she instinctively hadn't felt like going further with her G-spot experiments for a while.

In earlier chapters, we heard from women whose desires to become emotionally closer and more intimately connected in sexual relationships seemed to go hand in hand with their G-spot awakening, G-spot orgasms, and ejaculation. But some women's initial, excited attempts at exploration abruptly stop, or their eager enthusiasm turns to lethargy. This chapter will offer some explanations why this may happen. An effective approach for dealing with these blocks and restoring the healthy interest that allows a woman's process of discovery to continue is a G-spot massage, described in this chapter.

Since this method utilizes the most basic G-spot awareness techniques, like those explained in the "Stimulate Your G-spot" section in Chapter 4 and in Chapter 7, anyone from novice to expert can use the information presented here. Men will find important clues to the sources of diminished sexual interest in their partners, and an explanation of the important role they can play in helping their partner to overcome this obstacle.

Female ejaculation is not primarily about shooting ejaculate as far as you can, though that is fun. The G-spot is not about mind-blowing orgasms, though they are its luscious by-product. Rather, as we learned from sexologists and others in Chapters 2 and 6, G-spot awakening is about discovering that one's erotic body has infinite capacity to express emotions, love, and intimacy. Learning the G-spot's secrets is more about awareness than about technique, more about process than about goals, more about relaxation and nourishing oneself than adding another item to one's to-do list. When we approach the G-spot in this manner, we validate the power of the body and the feminine. Then we discover that the G-spot is our gateway to intimacy and our tool to express love.

☺ Sexual Trauma and the G-Spot ☺

The G-spot is a gateway to deeper aspects of sexual expression and intimacy that is entered by many women who are then stopped dead in their tracks by painful memories and events from their past. These women want to have sex with their partners and be open and trusting, but instead they feel an awful vulnerability that can end up causing distance and even rejection of the very people they seek connection with.

One out of four women experience a violent sexual crime during their lives. Even those who don't experience this type of trauma are negatively affected by living in a culture that attacks their bodies with pervasive and persistent messages like: "give me sex now—you don't have a G-spot—women don't ejaculate—let's do surgery to get rid of this female problem altogether and you'll feel better...." It is no wonder that women's sexual esteem and integrity can become seriously blocked.

These negative messages are stored physically, as memories, in the body. By understanding how this "body memory" operates, women can use a valuable physical technique that can help protect and heal them from all kinds of assaults to their sexuality, from minor to serious.

We hold emotional pain and physical trauma in the muscles and organs of our bodies. In the 1940s, Wilhelm Reich, a sexologist, psychologist, and student of Freud, theorized that there are circuits through which energy "streams" throughout the body. This energy can be blocked by emotional pain and trauma because these events are physically stored as memories in the muscles and organs, causing them to tense and/or cramp up, inhibiting the free flow of the energy streams. Reich called the creation of these muscular blocks "body armoring."

What are logical places for the emotional scars of sexual misuse or abuse to be stored? That's right, the G-spot and the PC muscles. For instance, rape is a traumatic event that can shatter the ability to open up and trust sexually, and it can create body armoring throughout a woman's genitals. This armoring may be why some areas on the G-spot are painful when touched. Unwanted, but permitted, entry into the vagina can also cause harm, because it requires "lies to the self" and disassociation between the mind and body. This, too, creates emotional scars that can lodge themselves in the G-spot, and manifest as areas that are numb to the touch.

Dealing with trauma is a new but growing field in psychotherapy. There are many good books that deal with the mental and behavioral effects of emotional pain and trauma, but few of them incorporate the healing that can occur by paying attention to the effects of trauma in the body. Psychotherapy is favorably assisted by massage. And for sexual trauma specifically, massage of the G-spot can be a beneficial aid to the healing process.

It is possible to reawaken the G-spot and heal emotional and sexual scars through understanding the capability of the G-spot to open up again to pleasure and energy. Over time, the G-spot naturally becomes more sensitive just through a growing awareness of it. This awareness creates other changes in behavior. You might ask your partner to slow down and wait until you are truly aroused. You will ask that they take time to enjoy and luxuriate in the sensuality and the emotions. You will notice the changes in your vagina when it feels more full, juicier, more sensitive. You may notice that you want your partners more. But I recommend giving the G-spot a little intentional assistance, to help unlock its full potential for pleasure. A G-spot massage is an excellent, effective way to do this.

⊚ Emotional Blocks to G-Spot Sensitivity ⊚

Before I explain the how-to of a G-spot massage, let me relate a story about my own foray into sexual healing using this powerful technique.

Some time ago, I was approached by Jerry, a massage therapist. He had seen my video about female ejaculation and wanted to tell me about his work with sexual abuse and G-spot massage. He was part of a small group of people doing this work and he invited me for a free demonstration.

I was intrigued, but I never did get a massage from him because I could not trust enough to let someone do this intimate research on me. Not even telling myself that the experience would be beneficial for my work with female ejaculation allowed my sensitive emotions to take him up on the offer. Years later, I met another sexual healer, Victor Gold, and even though I knew that I could trust him, I still was not ready to discover what painful secrets my G-spot held. So I let the opportunity with Victor go, too.

A year later, though, I began my own G-spot massage session, alone. I used the Crystal Wand (the slender Plexiglas sex toy discussed in Chapter 5) and felt around. I noticed a painful area on my G-spot. Touching it was highly uncomfortable. I put pressure on the spot for a couple of minutes and massaged the area, but kept some emotional distance. I did this a couple of times over the course of a few months. It felt like my G-spot was becoming fuller and more sensitive, but I wasn't sure. I did notice, however, that this area on my G-spot eventually stopped hurting.

A few months later, I decided to use another approach in one of these exploratory sessions with myself. I chose an obsidian gemstone in the shape of a dildo. I had decided to experiment with sexual healing in general, rather than looking for sore areas on my G-spot. As I let the gemstone fill my vagina, I breathed and practiced expanding my body to receive all the pleasure that I could. I had been single for two years at the time, and spent one year completely without sex with anyone. I wanted to "clean out" years of outmoded sexual habits. On this day, I felt that I was not just exploring but also performing a ceremony to express my sincerity about changing some sexual patterns that no longer appeared to benefit me.

As I proceeded with this semiformal celebration, I wasn't sure exactly what I would do. Then a mental picture emerged of someone who truly loved me, who was looking into my eyes and loving me through pleasuring my body. I had always tried to keep sex and love separate, but now I wanted to feel this sexual and loving pleasure in both my body and my heart. I wanted to feel what it was like to have my heart involved in the sex act, to have the warm feelings of love and the wonderful feelings of sex all mingled together. So I went with that mental image.

It was difficult to keep my erotic focus as I juggled thoughts of this person, my heart, his giving me love, my feeling love, and erotic pleasure all at once. I felt like a teenager learning to drive a stick-shift car. When I couldn't manage all this juggling and the feeling faded, I stopped, regrouped, and tried again.

Eventually, I managed to hold all these pieces together through an orgasm. It was so lovely, so warm, and so intense! But instantly afterward, I was overcome with the deepest sense of utter devastation I have ever felt in my life. I was reeling. The sense of loss of self, of void, of violent, laid-bare wasteland was so overwhelming that it consumed me. I was terrified and I felt I would not make it through: I would be destroyed. It felt like death. These are the feelings of trauma, and I had unknowingly triggered a trauma from my past.

I was able to get through this shock using therapy techniques I had already honed through practice. I journaled. I used affirmative "self-talk." I sang to myself. I moved my body. I even remembered to focus my eyes very intently on an object in order to center myself in my current reality. Slowly, I began to feel more grounded; the shattering emotions that had taken over my sense of reality so overwhelmingly fell away, and I came back to my present-day life and self. The dangerous darkness passed in fifteen minutes. But it left me shaken for two days afterward: I had exposed to the light a gaping wound in my psyche, one that had remained undoctored for years.

~ *Something to Remember* ~

Note that even though the sexual healing experience I describe in this chapter was one I undertook by myself, it is a good idea to approach sexual healing sessions with a person you trust. This person might be your lover, a trained sexual healer, or a psychotherapist. In this chapter, I describe G-spot massage, a sexual healing technique, being performed by a woman's partner as well as by a professional. Remember that you are not alone in your quest for healing; if you want to have somebody with you on this path, you should.

Certainly not all G-spot healing sessions will go, or need to go, this deep. One can avoid re-experiencing a trauma, especially all alone, as I later learned from my teacher Jwala, and it is best to do so. In the story at the end of this chapter, I describe a sexual healing session in which Jwala beautifully demonstrates how to sidestep this fall into the void yet still experience the healing that occurs when such issues are faced and brought to the surface. But if you find yourself in the predicament I did, or choose to go that far, there are some self-rescue measures you can use to guide yourself back to safety. If you start to experience overwhelming emotions when exploring your G-spot, whether alone or with a partner, take care of yourself by doing some or all of the following things:

1. Acknowledge your emotion to yourself. You can write about it, dance, play music, draw, garden, or try whatever "emergency" expressive measures work for you.

2. Ground yourself physically. Eat chocolate, meat, something sugary, or any comforting food. (This is not a time to worry about your health-food diet.) Drink warm herbal tea and avoid caffeine.

3. Protect your privacy. If you'd rather be alone, do not let anyone into your raw, cathartic space until you have recovered your bearings. Once you feel ready, call a trusted friend who will listen and be completely understanding and supportive.

4. Take notice of your surroundings. Focus your eyes on an object, willing yourself to be in the present moment. Remind yourself that the incident is in your past.

5. Make loud sounds and large, sweeping movements with your body.

6. Breathe slowly and rhythmically from your stomach.

7. Talk to yourself, using positive, affirming statements. Panic is triggered by negative thoughts, so avoid them and replace them with positive affirmations, images, and memories

8. Remember these feelings will pass. I assure you: *You will be okay.*

Specifically, this experience showed me how profoundly loving another person is connected, for me, to the devastating loss of my sister in childhood. Though years of therapy had made me aware of this, I had no idea how deep and terrifying the emotional devastation I felt after her death had been. I realized that I'd lost not only my sister, but also the loving comfort of my parents, who were also devastated. I was only six when she died and I can't consciously remember how I felt then. I had never realized how accurately my body had stored the experience. I had no inkling that these emotions were stored in my sexuality, wrapped up with it, and connected to my perceptions of myself and my ability to show love and accept it from others. But emotions from trauma exist outside of time. When triggered, they are experienced as if the incident happened only yesterday.

My next, and last, self-healing session was a year later. I chose the Creator as my visualized partner, and was rewarded with feelings of total union, utter love, and ecstatic bliss. My orgasm was long and shuddering, and the afterglow made my body vibrate with a joy that spread and settled into a vast sense of peace, lasting for many days.

Such bliss was my reward for facing a terrifying void, the shadow of deep-seated emotional trauma—facing Kali, as the Hindus call the goddess of destruction. I had gone on what some shamanistic traditions call a "soul retrieval." Why would anyone want to go through this emotional rollercoaster? Many people avoid the process and think those who attempt it are a bit crazy. But it is the best kind of therapy, for treating and bandaging psychological wounds left festering for decades. For myself, I only have to think of the ecstasy that resulted when I cleared the emotional blocks preventing me from accepting love, and of the joyous deepening of physical pleasure and emotional well-being experienced by others who have traveled this road, to be convinced of the value of this process. Seems worth it to me.

⚅ Give and Receive a G-Spot Massage ⚇

G-spot massage uses a finger (your own or somebody else's) or a sex toy to apply pressure to the G-spot, utilizing the same basic techniques described in Chapter 4 and Chapter 7. The purpose of this type of massage is to locate and remove the blocks to erotic pleasure stored as numbness or pain in the G-spot, and replace them with sensations of erotic, physical pleasure.

Although you can do a G-spot massage alone, as I did in the story above, the support of a partner has important benefits. A partner can provide a feeling of safety and help guide and ground the process. Having a real human being present, instead of the imaginary one I invited to my first session, helps re-establish trust, the damaging of which is a primary cause of emotional blocks. Later in this chapter I explain how to locate professional sexual healers who can also assist you through a sexual healing session.

Not all G-spot massage sessions have to deal with deep emotional issues. You can use them effectively for G-spot exploration, teaching your partner your "erotic map" and awakening your body to G-spot pleasure. Whichever purpose you choose, learning how to do a G-spot massage with a partner will help clear your sexual energy and let the love—as well as your ejaculate—flow.

In a G-spot massage session, the woman is the receiver and the person giving the massage is the supporter. Each role has certain responsibilities. The receiver should allow her sensations and emotions to flow and communicate what she is feeling to the supporter. The supporter should follow her instructions without judgment and without taking them personally, or as criticism. Nor should the supporter feel inadequate because he or she is doing only what the receiver requests: As the supporter you are supplying what she needs and has directly requested.

THE RECEIVER'S ROLE

As the receiver, your job is

1. to schedule uninterrupted time for the session.

2. to ask for whatever you need to be completely comfortable.

3. to open yourself to receiving pleasure and trusting the supporter.

4. to maintain eye contact with the supporter.

5. to breathe and relax.

6. to communicate clearly and directly what you are experiencing and how you want the supporter to touch you, in other words, to guide the supporter using your erotic map.

Relax and get comfortable, and prepare to feel whatever comes up. Open and relax your body, so that it can contain more pleasure, by breathing slowly and deeply. The breath carries pleasure from your genitals into other areas of your body, so you can literally hold more pleasure. It's like opening pores all over your body. Your body can become one large sexual organ, alive with sensual awareness and pleasure, if you choose to develop this ability over time. (Consult the Resources section for more information on breathing techniques for increasing sexual energy flow.) For these sessions, simply remember to breathe slowly and deeply and be conscious of your breath throughout the session.

THE SUPPORTER'S ROLE

As the supporter, your job is

1. to provide a warm room, a comfortable bed, soft lighting, and a quiet, distraction-free environment.

2. to focus your attention on your partner. You cannot ask her to "hold that thought" while you jump up and do something else. You must be 100 percent present for her.

3. to give freely of yourself.

4. to listen and acknowledge her with genuine feedback that reflects back to her what she has just told you and nothing more. You do not need to, and must not, come up with solutions to fix her "problem."

5. to look into her eyes and help her to keep looking into your eyes.

6. to remind her to breathe while you caress her body.

7. to apply her erotic map techniques when she requests that.

Remember that a healing-focused G-spot massage, versus a pleasure-oriented one, is not about making love. This is a healing session and is not intended to satisfy sexual needs. Rather, the supporter's role is to facilitate the receiver in an emotional process that has erotic, physical components. You will be rewarded for giving your time and energy in this manner with her increased ability to receive and feel pleasure when you do make love.

THE MASSAGE

The session begins with the receiver communicating to the supporter what physical touch turns her on. The supporter follows her instructions, asking her for feedback: "Slower? Softer? Does this feel good?" As the supporter performs what the receiver requests, he spreads the aroused sexual energy around her body by caressing her stomach, breasts, face, arms, and thighs. Both supporter and receiver maintain eye contact, and the supporter reminds her to slowly breathe in the sensation of pleasure. Once the receiver feels adequately aroused and emotionally comfortable to want the supporter to enter her vagina with a finger, she communicates this. At this point, the G-spot massage begins.

As the G-spot massage begins, the receiver identifies her physical sensations and stays present with any uncomfortable or pleasurable feelings. She should let go, clear her mind, and see what emotions arise, if any. She should notice what she is feeling in her body. Is one area ultrasensitive or painful? Is there an area that feels pleasurable? Does she feel nothing at all? The G-spot may actually be quite numb, or feel basically okay so that the strokes feel good, save for a sore spot or two. The receiver should communicate to the supporter about these emotions and sensations.

The supporter, in turn, stays connected via eye contact with the receiver, while applying firm and steady pressure to the area the receiver has identified. The supporter makes a mental note of which areas are pleasurable and which are numb or painful, and applies slow, circular motions to each area of the G-spot, while the receiver relaxes into the touch and breathes.

Numb or painful areas represent blocks to be removed. The combination of firm touch to the problem area on the G-spot and communication about any accompanying emotions can help restore pleasurable sensations to the problem area. The supporter does this by applying firm, steady pressure to the area and by encouraging the receiver to maintain eye contact and breathe slowly and deeply. The receiver assists in the removal of this block by staying present with any uncomfortable feelings and noting, out loud to the supporter, what emotion she is experiencing ("That feels like rage, or sadness, or joy"). As the receiver experiences an emotion, the supporter tries to keep mild pressure on the spot that triggered the emotion. The supporter should continue to massage the spot, and seek answers to these questions from the receiver: Is the area numb? If it is no longer numb, has it become painful?

If the receiver feels nothing. The supporter should discontinue the circular motions and should instead apply firm pressure all around the G-spot. Remind her to breathe and relax. Make a mental note of the receiver's emotional state at each place. She might feel frustrated, angry, depressed, lethargic, hesitant, or silly. Tell her to accept these feelings and breathe in. Tell her to breathe out relaxation and see if the emotions or physical sensations shift.

If the receiver feels pain. The receiver should breathe and visually relax her G-spot and PC muscles as the supporter presses firmly on the painful area. Notice if any emotions well up, such as sadness, longing, hurt, loneliness, or despair. The supporter can begin circular motions. Notice if the sensation becomes more painful, less painful, disappears, or becomes pleasurable.

If the receiver feels pleasure. The supporter should note the area on the G-spot where this pleasure is and try to find it the next time. Notice if it moves from place to place on her G-spot and experiment with pressure and motion. The receiver should continue to breathe and relax, noticing if the pleasure increases or decreases, and noting if feelings such as joy or intense sexual desire, vulnerability, happiness, or laughter arise.

The receiver should notice her reaction to these rising emotions:

1.   Did you tell the supporter to stop quickly? If so, you have shut down. This means you are not ready to feel what is going on, but that in itself is knowledge. When you are ready, you can go back and face what is there, waiting to be released and acknowledged.

2.   Did you feel nothing at all, become lethargic, or gradually lose interest in this exercise? This type of response is another kind of shutting-down mechanism, and may mean you are not ready to deal with what is there. Try again when you feel ready.

3.   Did you feel an emotion and note it, and then notice it pass? This type of response is a good release of blocked energy. Ask the supporter to continue to massage the area and notice if the sensation becomes more pleasurable.

4.   Did the emotion feel like it would utterly engulf you or that it could no longer be contained? This means that you are ready to acknowledge the emotion and learn what it has to tell you. It may flood furiously and overtake everything in its path, but hang on. However frightening the ride, however certain you are that the emotion will pull you under and threaten your being, you will surface. Floods are inherently cleansing, and that is what is taking place.

The receiver communicates when the uncomfortable sensation and emotions are passing, and the supporter asks if it is okay to continue to press and rub on the area. When the receiver agrees, the supporter begins making circular movements on the area. The supporter can attempt to stimulate pleasure to the area by alternately touching the area that has caused the distress and then touching a pleasurable area.

The supporter should notice if a painful area has become hot to the touch. If it feels hot, the block is being released, so it is good to ask the receiver if she is beginning to feel twinges of pleasure. If the receiver is beginning to feel pleasure, the supporter will know that the block has been removed or is being transformed.

The session can end there, unless the receiver wishes to proceed to another area. It is not necessary to proceed to an orgasm, but if the area feels pleasurable and a woman previously hasn't been able to feel erotic pleasure in the area, or in her G-spot as a whole, she may wish to progress to experiencing what there is to feel. This may lead to an orgasm, or it may not.

Intercourse is, of course, not the goal here, but can be appropriate if the receiver has problems with trust during intercourse, and the supporter is her sexual partner, and she would like to work on these issues together. (Erotic stimulation with fingers will also help with this issue.) Then, if the supporter is willing and able, you can proceed with penetration. Men should use their penis as they used their fingers, slowly stimulating her G-spot. The supporter should watch how it affects her, and hold still when emotions arise, keeping eye contact, reminding her to breathe and make eye contact, and to vocalize her sounds. Men who have mastered ejaculation control should use it now—it will aid you greatly in carrying out this part of your role in a G-spot massage session. Remember that, even with this level of intimacy in the massage session, the supporter is not the lover, but the healer.

Breathing deeply, keeping eye contact, voicing feelings, and remaining still can allow a powerful emotion to pass without having to re-experience the past event that caused it. It is often enough to feel the emotion, acknowledge it, and let it go. Sometimes the receiver will go deeper into the emotion. But however deeply she chooses to experience the process, the G-spot massage will tell a lot about the state of her erotic energy and emotional health.

⊚ Sexual Healing Anecdotes ⊚

Two women shared with me what they learned about their sexual wounds and how awakening their bodies to ejaculation helped them to overcome their wounds. After reading about my female ejaculation workshop, Meryl, an artist friend, shared her experience with me:

> I entered your workshop, feeling escorted in with the other women as I read your words, and before I knew it I was being coached right along with the others. I have spent a small amount of time meeting my G-spot over the past years but had always taken the shortcut to clitoral climax. This time I stayed there. I felt like I was chasing myself—like my G-spot was still being sat on by my father and his dominance and his abuse of me. Like he owned it, and I had to call to it behind him using my finger to feel and rub and probe. I had to link myself to my G-spot against his will, and not let his will deter me or cut me short. I listened to you tell me to stay there and not stop. And before I knew it, the link was stronger than the resistance that has deterred me all my life. Before I knew it, I reached the point of no return, and voilà! The waters flowed and I was astonished!
>
> I am looking forward to continuing this new experience. I want to learn the map home to myself. I want to understand it completely. I want my relationship to my own body restored 100 percent. And I know beyond a shadow of a doubt that this is the road I will take back to myself.

Holistic health practitioner and licensed massage therapist Dr. Corynna Clarke has been facilitating sexual healing in couples and individuals for many years. She draws from her studies in psychology, Eastern philosophy, Tantra, and the ancient Hindu traditions of the Dakini temple dancers in developing her methods. Being interviewed for the sacred sex part of my video *Tantric Journey to Female Orgasm: Awaken Your G-Spot,* she recounted her journey to an awakened G-spot and female ejaculation and what she learned about her innate ability to connect to a higher energy through a sexually healing cleansing process. She says:

> I had issues and wounds around sexual abuse. I numbed or shut down and could not stay present during sex. I couldn't feel pleasurable sensations. I felt there was more going on than I was experiencing. So I sought out a teacher with the intention of awakening and healing myself without the pressure of macho male attitudes.
>
> I've ejaculated pain and I've ejaculated a lot of sexual excitement. Mostly it's about intimacy with my partner. If I'm in a really beautiful, safe, and open space with him, then I can ejaculate. If I'm really moved, I emit spontaneously. If I push out my ejaculate, then I short-circuit the energy. If I do a gentle pushing, lean into it, then that extends the feeling of ejaculating. If I push, I get more distance but less sensation. When I was learning, I got too consumed in the pushing and not in the experience.
>
> Ejaculating is cleansing and erotic. The emotional aspect is like a deep surrender. I feel my energy more. I get high. After ejaculating and orgasming three or four times in one session, I become sensitive to my environment, in tune and centered. The orgasmic energy feels more like a healing throughout my body, akin to the higher healing of Goddess love or a state of bliss.

Wilhelm Reich said that because the body "streams" energy, people are capable of experiencing orgasmic sensations throughout their bodies. He called this a full-body orgasm. He went so far as to say that, in fact, a person's ability to experience a full-body orgasm was directly connected to that person's emotional health.

If you wish to go further in your explorations of G-spot massage and awakening your sexual energy flow, I recommend Margo Anand's thoroughly researched book, *The Art of Sexual Ecstasy.* This talented workshop leader, who holds a master's degree from the Sorbonne in France, developed techniques based on Reich's theories of body armoring and the theories of Alexander Lowen, the father of bioenergetics. She mixes these with the Tantric approach to sexual union, guiding the reader through the physical and spiritual realm of full-body orgasms.

It is a good idea to use G-spot massage to take a close look at the wellness of your G-spot, especially if you wish to experience all of its emotive, pleasurable, and spiritual capabilities and expand your intimate connections with your partner. Considering that men and women have been unaware of this component of a woman's sexual anatomy, and since sexual interactions aren't always engaged in with integrity, the G-spot could probably use a little special attention. Fortunately, there are a growing number of professionals helping women to heal this under-appreciated and often-wounded area of a woman's sexual anatomy.

◌ The Birth of the G-Spot Massage ◌

A growing group of professional massage therapists apply massage techniques to body-armored areas of the G-spot. Their aim is to release tension and heal emotional traumas that block or distort the flow of erotic pleasure. Modeled on integrative bodywork techniques, like those developed at the Esalen Institute in California in the 1960s and 1970s, massage is seen as a therapeutic aid to healing psychological problems. These genital massage techniques began to appear in the late 1970s.

Massage therapist and author Kenneth Ray Stubbs, Ph.D., held a faculty position at the Institute for the Advanced Study of Human Sexuality in San Francisco in 1977, where he designed a training program in sensate therapy. This led to the development of G-spot massage techniques, which he illustrated in his book *Erotic Massage: the Touch of Love* and in his *Erotic Massage I* and *Erotic Massage II* videos, which were published in 1989.

Joseph Kramer, Ph.D., a former Jesuit, developed the Taoist Erotic Massage (TEM) method in response to the AIDS epidemic that was affecting the gay male community in the early 1980s. TEM integrates Reich's "streaming of energy" concept with Eastern Taoist-based philosophies. In 1984, Kramer founded the Body Electric School in Oakland, California, where he instructed gay men and other practitioners in this method, which combines manual genital stimulation with breathing and massage. Practitioners hold their breath as long as possible while clenching every muscle in the body. All the erotic energy raised courses through the body as if a dam has broken, unblocking places of deeply repressed pain or other "impermissible" feelings. Kramer's practical, hands-on applications were presented in the video *Fire on the Mountain* (1992). He expanded these techniques into prostate massage for men, which he presented in the videos *Uranus: Self-Anal Massage for Men* (1996) and *Exploring the Land Down Under* (1993). Kramer later joined forces with erotic performance artist Annie Sprinkle, and they developed a set of G-spot massage techniques, which they later published in 1999 in the video *Fire in the Valley: An Intimate Guide to Female Genital Massage*.

Isa Magdalena was one of the first massage practitioners to train at the Body Electric School, where she was asked to tailor the technique to women. In her article "Celebrating the Body Electric for Women," she observes that women benefit from different methods than men:

> When I adapted Kramer's TEM for women, I found that women are not, in the first place, interested in genital exploration and arousal, even though their fear and excitement often seem to balance each other out. Instead, what comes first and foremost is permission to be friends with one's own body and feelings. There seems to be more hunger for nurturing touch—for example, whole body attention, which we receive so little of in daily life. Therefore, there is less focus on the TEM than in the men's workshops.
>
> Men, in general, love to be touched on their genitals and allow that easily. Women approach such an adventure with considerably greater apprehension. Yet, when we end the workshop with the TEM, there is

a breakthrough for most women, who get to experience their sexual power in a very different way than ever before. As much as I talk about the spiritual side of this work, I am convinced that the main healing and empowerment happens through reclaiming our bodies and our plain sexual pleasure. It is this that has been stolen from us, and it is [here that] we can find our connection with our spirituality.

In 2003, Kramer developed an online school called New School of Erotic Touch and a new video, *The Best of Vulva Massage,* which develops further the important elements involved in genital healing.

In the mid-1980s, workshop leaders and authors Charles and Caroline Muir of Source Tantra Institute in Hawaii and Margo Anand of Skydancing Institute in Colorado began to teach G-spot massage techniques in their workshops on sacred sex. In 1998, I wrote, directed, and produced the first video to feature a G-spot massage session, *Tantric Journey to Female Orgasm: Awaken Your G-Spot.* The video features Jwala, a student and teacher of Tantra since the mid-1960s and author of the book *Sacred Sex: Ecstatic Techniques for Empowering Relationships,* and Victor Gold, a Tantric practitioner.

I had a great chat over the telephone with Suzie Heumann, founder of Tantra.com, the premier Internet site for information and products relating to sacred sex, and she told me of her experience after taking one of the Muirs' workshops:

The very first time I ejaculated, I was in a weeklong workshop in Hawaii, and had spent the evening being filmed as a demonstrator in a segment of one of the Muirs' films on Tantric technique which had been shot that night. When my husband and I returned to our hotel room that evening, we made love, and I decided to mimic the weird sounds I had heard Caroline Muir make during lovemaking while doing the film. Well, the minute I opened my mouth, my whole body opened up and I ejaculated! It's like when you open the throat; your body can't hold onto anything—including ejaculate! It's amazing how making sounds is so important to achieve deeper orgasms because it opens up the energy in the body. I always encourage everyone to make sounds during sex!

Jack Painter, a psychologist in Marin County, California, and founder of the International Center for Release and Integration, developed a system of integrative bodywork that enables sexual energy release and does not involve genital massage. Instead it uses regular massage, breathing, and role playing, among other things. Called the Pelvic Heart Integration technique, it is featured in the video *Pelvic Heart Integration,* Tape II (2002), produced by Deborah Anapol of the Sacred Space Institute, also located in Marin County.

Integrative massage therapists, or bodyworkers as they are also called, differ from masseurs because of their training in psychology as it relates to the body. Masseurs understand the benefits of increased circulation and are trained in muscular anatomy but not in psychology or emotional release work. Masseurs are, therefore, unqualified to deal with the emotions (and in some cases, the traumas) that can be re-experienced when blocked energy that has long been stored in the body is finally released.

Bodyworkers and therapists, who understand the benefits of sexual healing to body, mind, and soul, come primarily out of the Tantra tradition. Together with sexologists, gay men and lesbians, and people who have worked in the sex entertainment field, they are developing and providing these techniques to those in need of healing. I admire their courage in providing badly needed services in spite of the risks posed to their personal freedom and financial security by laws that don't recognize the healing nature of this work.

"Sexual healing" is not yet a licensed field, though that by no means indicates that its practitioners are untrained or unqualified. In the Resources section at the back of this book, I have listed a few sources that can help you to locate a sexual healer specialized in working on trauma to the G-spot. Ask your gynecologist for further information on this essential therapy for sexual trauma recovery. Be advised, though, that although many doctors are becoming aware of sexual healing and its relationship to medicine, yours may not yet be. Judith Orloff, M.D., recognizes the value of sexual healing and discusses it in her book *Dr. Judith Orloff's Guide to Intuitive Healing: Five Steps to Physical, Emotional, and Sexual Wellness.* She has lectured to doctors across the country on its benefits, and in her book she reports that medical professionals, especially gynecologists and urologists, are interested in learning more. As one doctor told her, "Drawing on my sexuality is both a missing piece in my own growth and a part of patient care I've been searching for." Dr. Orloff deserves our gratitude for risking her professional credibility to broach a subject to her colleagues that the medical profession historically has shunned.

INTERVIEWING A SEXUAL HEALER

As in any profession, some practitioners are better trained and have more energy and enthusiasm for their work than others. As you would with any other kind of therapist, interview them before you begin any kind of treatment. What is their background? Their education? How long have they been doing this work? Why do they do it? What will they teach you? What is the process, and how long will it take? The answers you receive will give you a good idea of whether you feel comfortable with this person and will receive the care you seek.

Most genital sexual healers cannot, at this time, work under the auspices of professional therapy, but if you already work with a therapist, you can tell her or him what has come up for you in bodywork sessions. Similarly, you can tell your massage therapist/bodywork practitioner about what you're working on in your therapy sessions.

I hope that if you ever get the chance to work with a professional sexual healer, you'll take advantage of it. I didn't, as I mention at the beginning of this chapter, but perhaps I can blame it on my age. I spoke with John Ince, founder of the Erosha Institute in Vancouver, Canada, who teaches training classes for sexual healers. He explained that there is both a gender gap and an age gap between men and women seeking these services:

> While there is a huge demand for Erosha-style services for men, we have tried but failed to attract female clients. Very few women will pay to receive genital pleasure at the hands of a stranger, even though he or she is skillful and caring. However, I was recently approached by a small group of women in their twenties who urged me to introduce the service because they claim that there

would be a large demand for it in their age group. In general, I've
found that people a generation younger than mine (I'm forty-nine)
are far less erotophobic than my generation.

Kudos to you younger gals!

Though I hadn't accepted my first offer of a sexual healing session, I
was fortunate to participate in one as an onlooker when I was a complete
novice to this type of healing work. While I was doing research for my
video *Tantric Journey to Female Orgasm: Awaken Your G-Spot,* Victor
Gold and Jwala let me observe one of their sessions, which used a combination of a tantric approach to sexuality and Reich's theories of body
armoring. Let's see what happened.

⑤ A G-Spot Massage Session ⑥

When I first met Jwala, I instinctively liked her. She seemed like a female
version of a jolly Buddha, bubbly, open, and kind. Her first words are
always, "What's going on with you?" and she doesn't want a simple, polite
answer. She wants to hear your process, where you are today, what you are
struggling with in general.

I understand this and can tell her. She listens and then tells me what's
going on with her. It's an easy, flowing exchange because I feel she is utterly
free of judgment and will have only supportive and informative things to
say back to me.

Her work in Tantra spans thirty years, starting when Tantra was first
introduced to America. She has given workshops to thousands of people in
many countries, and her own healing journey through her life is an inspira-
tion. Her ability to know her body, recognize her feelings, and deal with old
limitations is as highly honed a skill as that of professional athletes or
master musicians. She has spent her life practicing and teaching others how
to remove blocks and open their bodies to pleasure and love.

When she says that women need a lot of healing in this life, all of her
experience and insight is in the statement. Now going through the life-cycle
changes of menopause, she has asked her longtime friend and Tantric healer

colleague, Victor Gold, to help her do some work on her G-spot, because she has noticed that menopause is shutting down her sexual desires. She invited me to one of their sessions and let me, at the time utterly unfamiliar with this type of healing work, ask questions about it.

Jwala's room is artistically decorated with lush fabrics, pillows, statues, and selectively placed mirrors. Fabrics cover the ceiling and walls. The effect is that of entering a Moroccan tent, lavishly decorated, extremely cozy, and sensual. Victor sits cross-legged on the bed, and Jwala takes a seat astride him. Both are draped only in sarongs that easily fall open.

"This position facilitates sexual energy shooting up to the brain, from the lower chakra through the spine to the cerebral cortex," Jwala informs me.

"Why would you want your sexual energy to shoot up into the brain?" I ask.

"If you love sex, you'll really love it in the brain," I am told. I nod thoughtfully, not sure I completely understand, but feeling that that's okay.

"What is a chakra? Why should people want to know about this?" I ask.

"There are seven energy centers that go up the body, starting at the base of the spine and ending a few inches above the head," Jwala answers. "They are true erogenous zones. When they're cleared and spinning with their natural energy, the whole body is turned on and full of vitality."

She and Victor start to slowly swing their bodies from side to side to balance their male and female energies. It looks a little silly and ineffectual to me, so I ask, "Why would you want to do this if you are a 'Neanderthal' kind of guy and happy with yourself, and this appears rather strange to you?"

"All your cells are sex cells," says Jwala. "This means all your body is an erogenous zone. When you balance your energies with those of your partner, the cells become activated. You stimulate the sex energy and bring it up into the heart and head, and it spreads throughout the body. It's done with the breath and eye contact."

She tells Victor what feels emotionally safe to her, like gazing into his eyes to establish trust, which helps her to stay present emotionally and trust whatever will come up in the session. She tells Victor and me, "Since menopause, my erotic feelings are now more hidden, and I must begin to feel pleasure before he can go into my G-spot to work on it."

"Why do you need sexual pleasure if this is a healing session?" I ask.

Victor explains, "You need sexual pleasure to stimulate sexual energy. But in this healing session, we send the sexual energy up and out to the whole body in order to clear the blocks of energy caused by body armoring. We can't clear the blocks with a quick sexual release and superficial stimulation, because that short-circuits our energy centers. Tantra teaches building sexual energy by delaying sexual pleasure, because then it runs all over the body."

He tells me a story of a woman who had twenty-five orgasms with a vibrator, then came to him because she still felt something was missing and didn't feel satisfied. "I told her to throw away the vibrator and start coming by delaying her pleasure."

"I'm going to spread the erotic energy all over her body." He begins to rub Jwala's thighs, stomach, breasts, and vulva.

Jwala explains her "erotic map" to Victor, telling him where and how she likes to be erotically touched. Then to me she says, "I learned my erotic map from my own exploration and an erotic massage workshop years ago."

"Are women's maps similar?" I ask, not really understanding the term. "No, you create your own." Then I get it. "Yes, of course," I think to myself, and understand that an erotic map is made up of the sites on your body that feel erotically good. Victor says, "One needs more time and conscious effort to circulate energy. Devote hours to making love! Make making love big and profound!" Victor is still rubbing her body all over.

Jwala teaches Victor how to stimulate her clitoris. I watch, fascinated, as she clearly directs him to do what feels best for her, and he listens, asks questions, and fine-tunes his technique, all without the slightest discomfort or affront. All the while, Jwala continues to breathe and relax, and they never break eye contact.

Jwala is now satisfied with her arousal level and tells Victor she is ready for him to enter her vagina. He inserts a finger slowly. "I like the window washer," Jwala says to him. "You want me to move my finger back and forth across your G-spot?" he asks, checking that he understood her request correctly. Jwala nods, and Victor moves his finger in the back-and-forth motion.

"A little harder, please," Jwala says. "Like this?" Victor asks. Jwala barely nods, and I can tell she is already not having a good time as he begins to work on her G-spot. "When you keep your eyes open and look at the healer, you can work through all kinds of sexual abuse," Jwala says, and begins to cry.

"Part of my sadness is I don't trust men. I keep looking at Victor's eyes to see the trust there, and that allows me to stay with my pain and fear and deal with them. If I close my eyes, I escape and don't deal."

Tears run down her face as she struggles to keep looking at Victor, while obviously wrestling with deep emotional issues. I feel moved and also strange, as if I am suddenly in a very sacred space; it's like the feeling of being present when great tragedy strikes another person. There is a sense of grief, but there is an undercurrent of otherworldliness and peace. I am fascinated and continue to watch her. It feels a little scary, a little too real. Also, I can't imagine accessing my feelings this quickly or understanding them so clearly. I feel awed by her skill.

"I feel rage now," she says to Victor and me. "This is a very wounded area. I can only take this in small doses, and I must breathe it out with every exhale, otherwise the rage overtakes me and I don't want to go on."

Victor says to me that if Jwala did that, it would end the session. "But transforming this pain into pleasure creates the healing. She is getting rid of armoring by releasing the psychic wounds of life. She must stay present with the emotion, ride it without getting swallowed up, and break through to the other side." His finger has stopped moving and he sits still. I notice his face wash over with empathy, but he does not reach out to comfort her. He keeps his eyes locked on hers.

I interject another question into this delicate moment, "How is this interaction occurring in a healer mode versus a lover mode?" Jwala responds, "Love, pleasure, and sexual fulfillment are what I get from my lover. This healing space is a place to release my wounds and heal my spirit." Victor nods and says, "Planetary healing starts with healing the wounds between man and woman. When two come together in sexual union, it creates a third energy, sometimes a child, sometimes something creative, or…. 'When two or more are gathered together in my name, I will be there.' "

I bite my lip and consider this. I guess I have heard this before, maybe in Sunday school.

"Energy moves," Victor continues. "It hits a block, and it stops. When the block gets released, it moves again. If it stays blocked, it gets reflected...." Jwala finishes his sentence, "...in being bitchy, naggy, frustrated."

Victor grins. "Many women get wounded sexually when they don't allow themselves to say no to sex when they really aren't in the mood, or when they succumb to heavy persuasion, or are forced into sex they do not want or welcome. These wounds are their hot spots. Literally, hot spots on the G-spot!" He lays his head on her abdomen and continues to work on her G-spot. Jwala lets out another wail.

"Why are you touching her stomach?" I ask, just to see what he will say.

"To be touched is grounding, and you feel safe. I put my head on her abdomen and my hand on her heart when she cries."

"I'm feeling tremendous energy in my arms," Jwala says. I marvel that Jwala can carry on a deep healing session and teach me at the same time.

"My finger is starting to burn. That is a sure sign that blocked energy has been released," Victor states excitedly.

"Why are you sitting so still now?" I ask him.

"Action facilitates. Stillness integrates the feelings she just got into touch with." They are both very quiet for a while. Then Jwala moans and starts a deep, rumbling roar. Jwala's sounds get very loud.

"You also release energy through loud sounds, and I, as facilitator, do, too, to show her I'm right there and present with her while she is experiencing this pain." Victor rumbles back at Jwala. They are like two tigers roaring at each other. I start to laugh.

Jwala tells me she has not ejaculated in a year because of menopause, and that she misses her juiciness. She asks Victor to keep massaging her G-spot, saying that she is feeling in the mood again. I watch as she changes, chameleonlike, from roaring pain to erotic pleasure. She uses loud sounds when she gets aroused, too, I notice. Thrashing wildly, moaning, screaming and yipping at times like a dolphin, she orgasms and releases a flood of ejaculate, laughing and thanking the Goddess for these gifts. Victor is smiling and nodding, still massaging her G-spot with his finger and "spreading the energy" around her body with his other hand. The sense of her emotional release is apparent and fills the room and there is a lovely clearing in her face. She looks ten years younger. I am infected by her joy and excitement.

Jwala is beaming. She just overcame her menopausal lethargy, and "cleared a few layers of mistrust and anger at men, too." I find it hard to disagree with that statement. She thanks Victor for "providing this space for women to heal and helping to bring back my juiciness." Victor removes his hands from her body, presses them together in a prayer position, bows at the waist, and says, "The pleasure was mine." Their countenances seem so sublime, I am reluctant to leave. But I thank them for letting me participate and quietly leave the room.

Eight years later, I can happily report that many of the techniques which felt bizarre at one time have now become commonplace to me. My sexual life does indeed feel imbued with more meaning and connection to my partner, and there are increasingly frequent instances of entering the same sacred place together.

In the next and final chapter, we'll take a brief look at what I truly hope will be the ultimate outcome of your G-spot and female ejaculation explorations: a dance with the higher sexual energies, where all longings find transforming satisfaction. From there, another world beckons, one beyond the scope of this book, but not beyond our imaginations or our abilities.

CHAPTER NINE

Connection to Self and Partner

◆

We hear a lot about how to keep the love alive in a relationship, doing every-thing from scheduling time for romantic getaways to trying stripteases, fantasy play, and fun sex toys. These approaches are definitely helpful. But, more importantly, as a woman's emotions get cleared and expressed through a gradually awakening G-spot, lovemaking oozes with potential to be juicier, more free, and more intimate.

You've got your G-spot stimulation techniques down, you've ejaculated, you're comfortable with emotions and the mess, you've cleared a few blocks, and found a partner who understands how your G-spot works and loves your ejaculate. What happens then? Fiery, intimate sex! Let's take a look at a love-making session that incorporates what we have learned so far about the G-spot and female ejaculation, and see how sexual intercourse with a pulsat-ing G-spot and flowing ejaculate can open the heart to connecting with your partner on a deeper level of intimacy, love, and caring—moving toward the reverence for each other embodied by sacred sex.

⊚ An Ejaculation Lovemaking Scene ⊚

Melissa heard Jack knock at the bedroom door. She took a deep breath, knowing he'd like the incense and alluring music drifting out to him, then glanced one more time in the mirror. The dark blue satin robe she'd chosen shimmered in the candlelight and set off the gold flecks in her auburn hair. Excited, Melissa took another deep breath and opened the door. He looked handsome to her! The scent of his muscular, freshly showered body was appealing and sexy. He presented her with three roses, each a different color. She smiled and thanked him. Jack kissed her tenderly on the cheek.

Melissa placed the roses in a vase by her bed, and they headed through the French doors to the subtly lit patio. Its centerpiece was a clawfoot bathtub she'd found at an estate sale two years before. Jack had helped her install it, raising it onto a sturdy wood platform. Earlier that evening she'd used the hose to fill it, and then added a mixture of rose and lavender oils to the warm water.

Jack led her to the edge of the tub. She let her robe fall to the ground and stepped into the bath, sliding to the bottom, up to her neck in the scented water. Jack took up a sponge and bathed her.

She inhaled deeply, relaxing into the light, sensuous, and soapy touch. His eyes sparkled with the thrill of her body and anticipation of their evening together. He enjoyed how she became putty in his hands when he teased her. Jack's slow and sensuous treatment aroused Melissa.

"Thank you for this," she said to him, still gazing into his eyes, cherishing his attentive touch.

He smiled confidently, gazing easily back at her. "Thank you for sharing your beautiful body with me," he said lovingly.

They kissed lightly and, it seemed to Melissa, forever.

After a while, she stood up, and he patted her body with a towel, kissing her as he went: her neck, her shoulders, each breast, her belly, clitoris, thighs, behind each knee, and the arches of her feet. He raised her arm and slid his lips up the side of her body until her fingers were drawn into his mouth.

She undid the drawstring on his pants and they fell to the floor. She bent to kiss his swollen penis, then led him inside to the bedroom. She poured massage oil into her hands, smiling at him as the musky scent permeated the air. He lay down on his stomach on the bed, and she straddled his smooth body. He relaxed at the feel of her erotic moistness against the rise of his buttocks, and she massaged his shoulders, neck, and back.

He turned over and she stretched out on his body. Their arms entwined, they synchronized their breath. She liked to feel him breathe out as she breathed in, and when she breathed out, he would breathe her in.

To Jack, it was like being lost in her cascading hair, and he felt intoxicated by their ritual of relaxation. His erection mellowed without concern; her excitement continued its slow climb. He sat up and crossed his legs and she straddled him. They traced the lines of each other's faces and stroked each other's hair, their gaze unbroken all the while. He patted her nipples, and gave each one a fond turn and twist, scratch and kiss. Melissa shuddered, and kept shuddering. She gently lifted his testicles taut and stroked them teasingly with her thumb, while in her eyes Jack saw a range of emotions run from humor to excitement to longing, and lastly, to love.

She sucked his nipple into her mouth, while he massaged her neck and breathed deeply to control his pleasure. It used to be so hard to stay in control with her, but these days, the breathing helped push the erotic desire out of his genitals and into his body. This relaxed his penis—for a while, anyway—until his desire returned with greater and growing fierceness.

He lay Melissa on her back, her head against the plush pillows. He was eager to lay his head between her thighs. Like arcs of golden love, they encircled him. He firmly pressed his lips between her urethra and vagina.

Melissa gasped at the touch of his mouth and moaned, full of longing and ache. She relaxed and completely gave herself up to his touch. She imagined her G-spot growing full and ripe and her ejaculate beginning to build. He caressed and kissed her vulva, until she desperately wanted him to touch her G-spot, yet she was grateful that he waited a little while longer for her heat to grow.

Jack withdrew from her satiny thighs, and knelt above her. He looked into her eyes, drawing small circles with a purposeful finger around her urethra and clitoris. He smiled as he deftly slipped his finger just inside her vaginal opening, as he knew what this would do to her, and he loved to give her pleasure. He drew his finger in and out slowly, many times, along the gutters of her G-spot. He pressed her G-spot's body and tail, rolling it around in his fingers, and Melissa moaned as if the very essence was being milked from her. He continued to stroke her G-spot and return her gaze.

Melissa's need mounted with this massaging of her G-spot. Sparks of energy, like rockets, cascaded down her legs, and she could feel the fullness of her G-spot refuse to let his finger go. His touch created a deep inner pool of pleasure that amazed her so, and oh, now this vaulting wave! As it crested inside her, she knew that her body was connected to his through his touch, unable to break away, suspended in time.

A long and earthy moan escaped Melissa's lips, her body beginning to coil and shake with pre-orgasmic pleasure. Breathing deeply, she felt the pleasure spread throughout her body, and she wanted more. She drew his throbbing penis to her mouth and sucked deeply, desire brimming inside her.

Jack yearned to nestle himself deeply inside the warm folds of her vagina. He had felt the swollen little gems in her G-spot, and knew that she was more than ready for him.

His penis full in her mouth, Melissa let it move gently back and forth over her moist lips. The last remaining tension left her body, which melted into buttery openness. There was nothing left of herself; she had given it all to him to enjoy, to use, to pleasure, to play with, and she relished the feeling of abandoning herself to him.

Jack withdrew his penis from her mouth, and led her out to the patio again to the edge of the tub. She turned and rested her hands on its rim, presenting her swollen vulva to him.

He entered her from behind with his penis, and his slow, steady, firm strokes felt huge to Melissa. She moaned, overcome by pleasure pulsating in every part of her brain, down to the very cells. Tiny bites of G-spot sensations cascaded from her full and sensitive G-spot down her legs and into her toes.

Jack could feel the pressure of her G-spot and its fullness on his penis. He could feel the rim of his penis stimulating it, slowly and deftly, over and over. Melissa's legs quivered. He covered her breasts with his hands, buried his face in her sweet-smelling hair, and sank himself deeply into her.

For Melissa, there was no lit courtyard, no room, no bodies; there was only Jack's presence, larger than life, and this growing wave of orgiastic warmth washing through her. She felt an utter loss of self and a delicious openness and receptivity to him. Bliss began to burst from her.

Her orgasmic contractions pushed his penis out of her, and a waterfall of ejaculate sprayed her thighs and his pelvis and ran in rivulets around their feet. She knew he loved it, and when he bent down to catch the drops with his searching tongue and thankful lips, she offered him another gush from her feminine spring.

She turned around to sit on the rim of the tub and grabbed for Jack, for more of him: deeper, harder, longer. He remained below the platform, for in this lower position, he could enter her easily. Melissa's head fell back in emotional and physical elation, as he jostled her very uterus, fast and deep inside her. Their love soared.

The boundaries of their being and everything around them dissolved, as if their identities had been transformed into pure light, love, and pleasure. Jack exploded in ethereal bliss as Melissa spun her orgasm out into union with Jack's love, which permeated her being, as her love permeated his.

Later, lying in bed, they embraced, holding each other for a long time, drenched in the feeling of peaceful union and floating in love.

◌ Tantra, Sacred Sex, and ◌ Female Ejaculation

The story above illustrates how the techniques that awaken the G-spot, by their very nature, can create more intimacy in a relationship. The techniques can open a door into the realm of sacred sex—the heart of a Tantric experience.

Many couples have expressed to me an interest in Tantra. In America, "Tantra" has become the code word, if you will, used by couples who want to bring sacred sexuality into their love life. Tantra found its way into American bedrooms largely through the success of Margo Anand's and Charles and Caroline Muir's teachings. Their workshops, books, and videos, for couples who seek to increase their communication and sexual intimacy skills, are styled on the ancient sexual-spiritual tradition of Tantra.

Tantra requires and teaches the important elements of sacred sex: connection with the heart in sexual union, complete comfort with the body, a high level of ability to communicate sexual needs, virtuosic skills in the art of sensuality, physical agility, awareness of how sexual energy feels when it runs through the body, and the willingness to enter a mystic state. Like any spiritual practice, the ability to integrate the teachings and enter higher and higher states of consciousness for longer and longer periods grows over time and with practice. (Basic Tantric philosophy and its views on female ejaculation were discussed briefly in Chapter 3 in the section "Nectar of the Gods—Ancient India.")

A vast and uncharted realm of sacred sex awaits couples who wish to experience the wisdom of Tantra; use the Tantric approach for expanding connection, pleasure, and love; and feel an energy flow that connects them to the universal force. This level of sexual exchange offers an ease and degree of satisfaction with one's sexuality that many individuals yearn for.

I interviewed David Steinberg, editor of the anthology *Erotic by Nature: A Celebration of Life, of Love, and of Our Wonderful Bodies*, for my video *Tantric Journey to Female Orgasm: Awaken Your G-Spot*. He recounted an experience he had when using a Tantric approach to erotic intimacy:

> I was with a woman once who was struggling to have an orgasm. I put all of my being, all of my conscious awareness, into the tip of my finger, very purposefully, and then put it inside her. It pushed her over the edge almost instantly. It was amazing! It's not a technique; that's misleading. Purposeful touch is about listening and following sexual energy, rather than always trying to lead it.

Steinberg continues by describing the rewards he found in sacred sex:

> I turn myself over to this heightened sexual experience, then start to go into the "oh, my goodness" of it; I go into another world. Everything becomes magical. Things light up and what lights it all is your own fascination.

He also expresses his thoughts on why sacred sex is practiced in few Westerners' bedrooms:

> Sex is approached too scientifically. [Sex manuals] are helpful, but make people think too technically and mechanically about sex. Joseph

Campbell, who studied the mythological stories and traditions of tribal cultures around the world, said that religion is not to be taken literally, and I would add that neither is sex. Addressing sex from a scientific perspective is fine, but the more profound stuff of sex is mystic, mysterious, and about wonder.

I'm reminded of the hundreds of men I talked to while dancing on their laps as an erotic performer, and I can see in my mind the pained faces of many of the women who attend my workshops and lectures, who yearn for "something more" from sex. For women, this "something more," as we discussed in Chapter 7, is a desire to acknowledge and satisfy their soulful approach to sexual attraction and arousal. For men, it is a painfully unmet desire to engage in erotic exchange with a woman who is sexually welcoming, free and loving.

Awakening female ejaculation and the G-spot can lead you through the realm of expanded erotic intimacy—soulful, connected, and juicy intercourse with another human being—and then into the lap of sacred sex and its mystic states of connecting, with, in, and through your beloved partner, to the universal Mind. If you wish to explore this experience, consult the Resources section at the back of this book for more information on sacred sex and Tantra.

⑤ The G-Spot Is Alive and Well ⑥

As I sat at my computer one quiet and sunny Saturday morning finishing up this book, I opened my e-mail to find a lone message from the Internet G-spot chat group. It said simply, "The G-spot is dead."

The message was obviously an offensive hit-and-run, but that morning it struck me as funny. I couldn't quite delete the message and forget about it, however; instead I stared at it awhile. I continued to alternately chuckle at and feel disturbed by this message periodically throughout the day. Finally, its significance occurred to me. "Yes, of course," I thought. "The G-spot *is* dead. That's why we can't find it!"

The message bolstered my resolve to finish this book, and affirmed its premise, that we can awaken the G-spot and the feminine ability to ejaculate. It reminded me why I was writing this book in the first place: to remove the obstacles that have stood in the way of experiencing and enjoying this feminine birthright.

Okay. The G-spot is dead. *And* now you've learned how to resurrect it and allow its ejaculate to flow freely forth!

⊚ **What You Have Learned** ⊚

WE KNOW THAT FEMALE EJACULATION EXISTS AND IS NATURAL AND NORMAL, BECAUSE ITS SOURCE, THE FEMALE PROSTATE, HAS BEEN SCIENTIFICALLY ESTABLISHED.

You have learned the reasons why the G-spot has been considered "dead" by most individuals, mainly because doctors have viewed it as a vestigial, nonfunctioning organ. You have also learned how scientists have proven that the G-spot does exist by studying it in exhaustive detail over the past two decades. You have learned that the female prostate has two primary functions: to produce and excrete prostatic fluid (ejaculate) and to provide the body with serotonin—and possibly other hormones.

You have learned some of the important properties of female ejaculate: Its glucose aids a supportive vaginal environment for sperm, thereby playing an important role in insemination; it may soothe and protect the urethral tract, thereby lessening bladder infections and urethritis (irritation of the urethra); and it possesses healthful minerals, such as zinc.

FEMALE EJACULATION CAN BE LEARNED AND CAN BE PHYSICALLY CONTROLLED.

You have learned that all women have the anatomy to ejaculate, because all women are born with a prostate. You have learned that ejaculation in both men and women can be controlled, and that some women unconsciously stop its release to the outside of the body, sending it, retrograde, into the bladder. You have learned that women can teach themselves to expel their ejaculate out of the body with or without an orgasm, and that the amount of female ejaculate can increase over time in most women, once their comfort with ejaculation increases.

You have learned many reasons why the flow of female ejaculate can be stymied or reduced: where a woman is in her menstrual cycle; the strength of the PC muscles; surgery in the pelvic area; the position a woman is in when ejaculating; negative attitudes or misinformation about what female ejaculate is; and the size of the prostate.

FEMALE EJACULATION HAS AN ANCIENT HISTORY.

You have learned that female ejaculate was known and honored as a sacred fluid by indigenous cultures in America, China, Greece, India, and Japan and in Africa, Europe, and the South Pacific. You have learned that most of these cultures considered female ejaculate healthful.

You have learned that female ejaculate was believed to contain essences essential to the creation of new life, and that it may have been part of a Celtic creation myth. You have learned that female ejaculate was believed to be a means for men to gain immortality, and that its energy is used by modern-day priestesses for rebalancing a damaged psyche.

THE G-SPOT CAN BE LOCATED AND STIMULATED AND ITS EROTIC MAP REVEALED.

You have learned that the G-spot is ramp-shaped in most women, and that it's usually located close to the urethral opening and surrounds the urethral canal. You have found the G-spot's head, body, tail, and gutters.

You have seen the G-spot, and watched it move as you used your PC muscles to push it out toward the opening of the vagina. You have watched the urethral opening move as well, as the vagina is penetrated. You understand that the urethra, which runs through the prostate/ G-spot, is an important part of the female sex organ, and that stimulation of it is erotic and pleasurable for many women.

You have learned how to stimulate your G-spot to build ejaculate fluid by rubbing, squeezing, and rolling the G-spot's body, tail, and gutters with your fingers. You have felt the G-spot swell with ejaculate due to this stimulation, and perhaps even felt the "little nodules" present in the G-spot when it is full of ejaculate. You have practiced variations on this stimulation technique with a G-spot sex toy and used the erotic map you created to communicate your G-spot stimulation discoveries to your partner.

THE G-SPOT PRODUCES A UNIQUE TYPE OF ORGASM.

You have learned about the G-spot orgasm. You have learned that the G-spot connects to a different nerve than does the clitoris, and therefore provides different orgasmic sensations. This G-spot nerve also stimulates the bulk of the PC muscles to contract during orgasm, which aids in ejaculation.

You have learned how to distinguish between three kinds of orgasms and how each relates to female ejaculation: the clitoral, the G-spot (blended), and the uterine orgasms. You have heard how other people experience these orgasms and how they do or don't ejaculate when they have them. You have learned techniques to practice the G-spot orgasm, how to begin integrating ejaculation into your orgasms, and the success you can expect to achieve when trying to ejaculate with each kind of orgasm.

THE G-SPOT IS BY NATURE ULTRA-SENSITIVE TO EROTIC TOUCH AND PRODUCES EJACULATE.

You have learned your G-spot's "erotic map," and that its sensitivity can grow over time with awareness and increased skill. You have learned how female ejaculation can be produced with G-spot stimulation, with or without an orgasm, and with or without a partner.

You have learned a bit about the nature of women's soulful approach to eroticism, how to ground this eroticism in the G-spot, and how to facilitate G-spot-awakening with artistic expression and with sex toys. You have learned some useful places to thoroughly enjoy a free flow of female ejaculate.

MOST MEN LOVE WOMEN WHO EJACULATE, AND WOMEN ARE ENCOURAGED WHEN THEIR PARTNER ENJOYS FEMALE EJACULATION.

You have learned that a partner's attitude toward female ejaculation can assist (or hinder) a woman's ability to ejaculate and can promote the relaxation necessary to let go and let it flow. You have learned how to tell a partner about female ejaculation and solicit help, and how to help a female partner learn how to ejaculate.

You have learned that male ejaculation control and mastering male multiple orgasms not only help a woman awaken the sensitivity of her G-spot but also take male sexual pleasure and satisfaction to a new level. You have also learned sexual positions that facilitate ejaculation as well as a deeper level of intimacy.

SEXUAL ENERGY CAN BECOME BLOCKED IN THE G-SPOT AND CAN BE RELEASED BY A G-SPOT MASSAGE.

You have learned that emotional blocks, caused by negative sexual experiences, can numb the G-spot or cause it to be painful, indirectly preventing female ejaculation. You have learned how to perform a G-spot massage to awaken its sensitivity and/or release these blocks, and how to deal with any strong emotions that may arise while performing this activity. You have learned a bit about the development of G-spot massage and the schools and healers who can offer instruction and guidance.

THE G-SPOT IS A GATEWAY TO INCREASED INTIMACY AND SACRED SEXUAL ENERGY EXCHANGE.

You have learned that the G-spot is a gateway to greater intimacy, and that using its sexual energy can open a door to experiencing a sacred, sexual exchange with a partner.

You have acquired many tools to help you understand female ejaculation and the G-spot, and I hope that you have already begun to use and experience them. They will create never-ending opportunities to develop your sexuality, which can keep your sexual life flowing with discovery for a lifetime. Therefore, if you are ready, don't delay!

⑤ **What You Can Do Now** ⑥

Awaken your G-spot. Use the G-spot stimulation explorations in Chapter 4, and the G-spot orgasm explorations in Chapter 5, to continue to practice, practice, practice becoming acquainted with your G-spot and how to build its ejaculate fluid. Learn everything you can about your erotic map.

Get your ejaculate waters flowing again. Use the attitude and muscle tests, the G-spot explorations, and the non-orgasmic ejaculation explorations in Chapter 4 to become familiar and comfortable with your feminine ability to bless yourself and your environment with your ejaculate. Use the techniques in Chapter 5 to ejaculate with an orgasm, as well as to experiment with G-spot sex toys and practice, practice, practice ejaculating!

Understand and experience G-spot orgasms. Use the continuum of G-spot orgasms, and the techniques that assist in creating G-spot orgasms, discussed in Chapter 5, to practice, practice, practice building awareness of what a G-spot orgasm feels like and its variety of sensations, and to build your skills at attaining the type of orgasm that aids your ejaculation response.

Share female ejaculation and your G-spot with your partner. Use the guidelines for engaging your partner in your desire to ejaculate presented in Chapter 6, and the sexual positions suggested there, to practice, practice, practice your new skills at ejaculating within the context of a sexual partnership. Use the G-spot massage session techniques in Chapter 8 to awaken your G-spot further and to develop communication skills that will assist you in guiding your partner to your pleasure spots.

Monitor your G-spot's physical and emotional health. Use the PC-muscles exercises in Chapter 4, and the G-spot massage techniques in Chapter 8, to keep your ejaculation muscles strong and flexible and your G-spot's sexual energy flowing freely.

Attempt a uterine orgasm and experience sacred sex with a partner.
Share your G-spot awakening with a special person and practice, practice,
practice experimenting with G-spot orgasms in order to experience a
uterine orgasm and the powerful connection of blissful sexual union.

Remember, female ejaculation is a choice. We choose to be who we are and
do what we want. Now, there is another sexual choice open to women and
their partners: the feminine waters of female ejaculation. Choose wisely,

~ A Word about the G-spot and the Female ~ Ejaculation—Awakening Process

Learning about the G-spot is not a linear process; it is circular. As your
G-spot becomes alive and the pleasures evolve, the circle is completed. Then
a new circle begins. You will get through the cumbersome first solo explorations and the equally cumbersome sexual positions. You will get through
the painful or scary emotional clearing of pent-up desires. You will have a
bliss experience. Then the process of discovering what your G-spot is capable of and how easily and fully your ejaculate can flow will begin all over
again, like peeling away the first layer on an onion, only to find another one
there to be peeled away. Enjoy each phase of the awakening, and please
remember: It is a long-term process.

The goal of exploring the G-spot and female ejaculation is the journey, the
process of discovery, not ejaculating or having a G-spot orgasm. The guiding
rules are to have fun while you learn and to trust the process. Take your time
learning how to stimulate your G-spot and how to ejaculate. Avoid becoming
discouraged and giving up. Rather, find your own unique expression and your
own physical capabilities.

enjoy your decisions, and remain responsible for them. You will likely discover that the following and other delights grow out of your explorations:

1. You find new pleasures with your clitoral orgasms.

2. "Sport sex" becomes even more fun and playful.

3. Ejaculating becomes easier.

4. You feel more variety in orgasms and sensations of pleasure.

5. You experience greater presence, openness, and satisfaction in your sexually intimate encounters with a partner.

6. You have your first "bliss" orgasm.

May your feminine ejaculate forever flow free, be joyously profuse, and be honorably acknowledged.

~ *A Female Ejaculation Blessing* ~

I bless all women courageous enough to take on this journey of awakening the soul of their femininity, bringing it back into our bedrooms and into our lives.

I bless all the men who take the time to understand the feminine soul and are willing to accommodate it by blending and changing.

I bless all the people who have studied female ejaculation, and those whose waters never quit flowing; may you lead and teach.

I bless society for accepting female ejaculation and honoring its deeper quality, not making it another trend or trivializing its deeper significance.

I bless the babies born in flowing ejaculate, for they will be truly welcomed into a new world.

I thank the Twisted Hairs for traveling around the world to bring us greater understanding and to show us how similar we all are.

I bless your sexual union; may it rise to new heights and enrich your lives.

I bless all the peoples of the earth, that they stop warring, open their hearts and minds to love, and honor the creative sexual energy in each one of us, an energy that is a reflection of the ultimate Creator.

Glossary

amrita—Sanskrit word for nectar, holy or blessed water, used in some contexts for female ejaculate

amaroli—Sanskrit word for the practice of taking *amrita*

amplexus reservaturs—a Latin term used to describe the practice of withholding ejaculate, in both men and women

apnea response—temporary suspension of breath, often encountered during a blended (G-spot) or uterine orgasm.

blended orgasm—the physical and emotional sensations and climax created by stimulation of both the clitoris and the G-spot; *see also* G-spot orgasm

body armoring—patterns of musculature or ways of holding he body that are created by energy streams in the body being blocked due to unreleased physical or emotional pain or trauma

chakra—Sanskrit term for six or seven energy vortices or centers located along the spine and neck from the tailbone to just above the head

chi—Taoist term for the subtle energy or life force in the body, called *prana* in Sanskrit

clitoral orgasm—the physical sensations and climax created by stimulating only the clitoris; does not facilitate female ejaculation

clitoral sponge—another name for the female erectile tissue network

clitoris—highly sensitive area of a portion of erectile tissue in women located on the outside of the vulva

ejaculate—fluid created by the prostate gland in both men and women, emitted during arousal

ejac rockets—sporadic, erotically pleasurable shooting sensations felt in the female genitals and legs during G-spot stimulation and arousal that can signal the onset of ejaculation

erectile tissue—network of tissue in the genital area that fills with blood and swells when directly stimulated or during sexual arousal

erotic map—a way of conceptualizing the erotic areas of a person's body, the types of touch a person most enjoys, and the duration of touch that is most pleasurable on these areas; unique to every person

G-spot—another word for the female prostate; includes the erectile tissue surrounding the prostate (urethral sponge)

G-spot orgasm—*see* blended orgasm

glucose—a sugar that makes up a part of the male and female ejaculate and creates a supportive environment in the vagina for sperm

Jade Cavern—Taoist term for the vagina

Kegel exercises—a set of biofeedback exercises designed by Dr. Kegel to strengthen the PC muscles to aid orgasm and ejaculation and reduce urinary stress incontinence

labia—the inner and outer "lips" of tissue at the entrance to the vagina

liquor vitae—Latin term for a life-enhancing essence that the Greeks and Romans believed resides in male and female ejaculate

lotus nectar—a Tantric term for female ejaculate

meatus—*see* urethral meatus or meatus prostate

meatus prostate—the most common type of female prostate; it is ramp-shaped and located near the urethral opening

myograph—a device used to measure the contractions of the PC and uterine muscles during arousal and orgasm

orende—Quodoushka term for a subtle, ethereal energy in the body (*see* chi)

PSA (prostate specific antigen)—the scientific "marker" that identifies prostatic fluid in male and female ejaculate

PC muscles—the *pubococcygeus muscles;* a set of pelvic muscles, including the uterine muscles, which aid ejaculation and cause the contractions in an orgasm

pelvic muscles—a group of muscles which includes the PC and uterine muscles

pelvic nerve—a nerve which serves the urethra, bladder, uterus, prostate, and the back two-thirds of the PC muscles

perineal sponge—a portion of erectile tissue, less dense than that found in the clitoris, which lies between the vagina and the anus

perineometer—a modern biofeedback device used to measure the strength and flexibility of the PC muscles and guide women in the correct practice of Kegel exercises

prostate—an organ of glands, ducts, and smooth muscle located in the wall of the urethral canal that creates and secretes ejaculate fluid in microscopic amounts at all times, and in noticeable and large amounts when sexually stimulated. The shape and location of the prostate varies in women, with the meatus type being the most common in the majority of women

pudendal nerve—a nerve that serves the clitoris, vulva, and front one-third of the PC muscles

prostatic fluid—the fluid created and excreted by the prostate; a major component of female ejaculate

prostate gland—*see* prostate

pubococcygeus muscles—*see* PC muscles

retrograde ejaculation—the act of releasing ejaculate fluid into the bladder rather than to the outside of the body

sex organ, female—defined in this book as the vulva, clitoris, urethra, vagina, prostate (G-spot), pelvic muscles and nerves, and erectile tissue

sex organ, male—defined in this book as the penis, testicles, urethra, prostate, pelvic muscles and nerves, and erectile tissue

sex toy—an object used for genital stimulation to achieve erotic arousal or orgasm

speculum—instrument used in the gynecologist's office or self-help clinic to open the vaginal walls in order to see the cervix

spongy tissues—*see* erectile tissue

Sanskrit—an ancient, written language of India

Tantra—an ancient Indian philosophy and spiritual practice that viewed the sex act as a means to cosmic union or universal consciousness

Taoism—an ancient Chinese spiritual philosophy and science

urethral meatus—the fleshy area of the vulva that surrounds the female urethral opening

urethral sponge—a portion of erectile tissue that surrounds the urethra and female prostate

uterine orgasm—the physical sensations created by the jostling of the cervix, stimulating the sensitive lining of the uterus

uterine muscles—a portion of PC muscles

vaginal muscles—another term for PC or pelvic muscles

vaginal orgasm—a rarely used, vernacular term for a G-spot orgasm

vestige, vestigial—generally used scientifically for a part of the anatomy that has no use yet resembles a functioning counterpart in the opposite sex

vibrator—a sex toy that vibrates and is used for genital or other stimulation

vulva—outer portion of a woman's genitals comprising the clitoris, urethral meatus, labia, and vaginal openings

water goddesses—Greek term for labia

yoga—Sanskrit term for "union"; an ancient Indian philosophy; a meditation practice that utilizes the breath and a system of physical stretches and held positions to encourage mental and physical control over mind and body

Yoni—Sanskrit term for the vagina and vulva

References

CHAPTER 1: A PEEK INSIDE A FEMALE EJACULATION WORKSHOP

Sundahl, D. 1994. "Battle Scars: Freeing Women's Erotic Voice." *On Our Backs* 10:1.

Sundahl, D.; "Stripper." In *Sex Work: Writings by Women in the Sex Industry,* edited by F. Delacoste; and P. Alexander. San Francisco, CA: Cleis Press, 1987.

CHAPTER 2: WHAT *IS* FEMALE EJACULATION?

Anand, M. *The Art of Sexual Ecstasy.* New York: Tarcher/Putnam, 1989.

Bell, S. "Liquid Fire." In *Jane Sexes It Up,* edited by M. L. Johnson. New York: Four Walls, Eight Windows, 2002.

Bell, S., and K. Daymond. *Nice Girls Don't Do It.* Toronto: Daymond and Bell, 1990.

Cabello, F. "Female Ejaculation: Myth and Reality." In *Sexuality and Human Rights: Book of Proceedings of the 13th World Congress of Sexology,* edited by J. Baras-Vass and M. Perez-Conchillo. Valencia, Spain: E.C.V.S.A., 1997, 325–33.

Cabello, F. "Are Our Ideas on Vaginal Lubrication Correct?" *Abstracts Book of the 15th World Congress of Sexology.* Paris, 2001, 31.

Cabello, F. 1998. "Female Ejaculation: New Biochemical Findings." *Revista Sociedad Argentina de Sexualidad Humana* 12(1):36–42

Chia, M. *Taoist Secrets of Love: Cultivating Male Sexual Energy*. Santa Fe, NM: Aurora Press, 1984.

De Graaf, R. 1972. "New Treatise Concerning the Generative Organs of Women (1672)." Translated by H. B. Jocelyn and B. P. Setchell. *Journal of Reproduction and Fertility* 17.

Dodson, B. *Sex For One: The Joy of Selfloving*. Westminster, MD: Harmony Books, 1986. Reissued New York: Three Rivers Press, 1996.

Fatale, F. 1992. "This Is What Fanny's G-Spot Looks Like." San Francisco, CA: *On Our Backs* 8:1.

Federation of Feminist Women's Health Care Centers. *A New View of a Woman's Body*, 2nd ed. Illustrated by Suzann Gage. Los Angeles, CA: Feminist Health Press, 1991.

Freud, S. *Basic Writings of Sigmund Freud*. Translated and edited by A. Brill. New York: Modern Library, Random House, 1938.

Gräfenberg, E. 1950. "Role of the Urethra in Female Orgasms." *International Journal of Sexology* 3:145–8.

Hooper, J., and D. Teresi. *The 3-Pound Universe*. New York: G.P. Putnam's Son, 1986.

Huffman, J. W. 1948. "The Detailed Anatomy of the Paraurethral Ducts in the Adult Human Female." *American Journal of Obstetrics and Gynecology*, 55:86–101.

Kinsey, A., et al. *Sexual Behavior in the Human Female.* Philadelphia, PA: W.B. Saunders, 1973.

Ladas, A., B. Whipple, and J. Perry. *The G-Spot and Other Recent Discoveries About Human Sexuality.* New York: Holt, Rinehart and Winston, 1982; New York: Dell, 1983.

Lessing, D. M., *The Golden Notebook.* Harmondsworth, U.K.: Penguin Books, 1964; New York: HarperCollins, 1999.

Perry, J. 1999. "Effects of Clitoral and G-Spot Stimulation on the Pelvic Muscles." Dr. Gspot's Website, www.drgspot.net.

Schubach, G. 1997. "Urethral Expulsions During Sensual Arousal and Bladder Catheterization in Seven Human Females." Doctoral research project, Dr. GSpot's Website, <www.drgspot.net>.

Schubach, G. 1997. "Bibliography of Female Ejaculation." Doctoral research project, *Electronic Journal of Human Sexuality* <www.ejsh.org/Volume4/schubach/abstract>.

Sevely, J. L. *Eve's Secrets: A New Theory of Female Sexuality.* New York: Random House, 1987.

Sevely, J. L., and J. W. Bennett. 1978. "Concerning Female Ejaculation and the Female Prostate." *Journal of Sex Research.* 14:1–20.

Singer, I. *The Goals of Human Sexuality*. New York: W. W. Norton, 1974.

Singer, J., and I. Singer. "Types of Female Orgasm." In *Handbook of Sex Therapy,* edited by J. Lo Piccolo and L. Lo Piccolo. New York: Plenum Press, 1979, 175–86.

Stifter, K. *Die Dritte Dimension Der Lust—Das Geheimnis Der Weiblichen Ejakulation* [*The Third Dimension of Lust: The Secrets of Female Ejaculation*]. Frankfurt: Ullstein, 1988.

Sundahl, D., and N. Kinney. *How to Female Ejaculate: Find Your G-Spot with Fanny Fatale.* San Francisco: Fatale Video, 1991. Re-edited: Sundahl, D. *How to Female Ejaculate: Find Your G-Spot with Deborah Sundahl*. Santa Fe, NM: Isis Media, 2002.

Whipple, B., and B. R. Komisaruk. 2002. "Brain (PET) Responses to Vaginal-Cervical Self-Stimulation in Women with Complete Spinal Cord Injury." *Journal of Sex and Marital Therapy* 28.

Zaviacic, M. *The Human Female Prostate: From Vestigial Skene's Paraurethral Glands and Ducts to Woman's Functional Prostate.* Bratislava: Slovak Academic Press, 1999.

Zaviacic, M. *The Human Female Prostate and Its Role in Woman's Life: Sexology Implications. 15th World Congress of Sexology,* Paris, 2001.

Zaviacic, M., J. Jakubovsky, S. Polak, A. Zaviacicova, I. K. Holoman, J. Blazekova, and P. Gregor. 1984. "The Fluid of Female Urethral Expulsions Analyzed by Histochemical, Electron Microscopic and Other Methods." *Histochemical Journal* 16:445–7.

Zaviacic, M., J. Jakubovsky, S. Polak, A. Zaviacicova, and I. K. Holoman. 1984. "Rhythmic Changes of Human Female Squamous Cells During Menstrual Cycle." *International Urology and Nephrology* 16:301–9.

Zaviacic, M., and R. J. Ablin. 2000. "The Female Prostate and Prostate-specific Antigen: Immunohisto-chemical Localization, Implications of this Prostate Marker in Women and Reason for Using the Term 'Prostate' in the Human Female." *Histology and Histopathology* 15:131–42.

Zaviacic, M., V. Jakubovska, M. Belosovic, and J. Breza. 2000. "Ultrastructure of the Normal Adult Human Female Prostate Gland (Skene's Gland)." *Anatomy and Embryology* 201:51–61.

CHAPTER 3: THE ANCIENT HERSTORY OF FEMALE EJACULATION

Anand, M. *The Art of Sexual Ecstasy.* New York: Tarcher/Putnam, 1989.

Chia, M. Personal correspondence with the author, 2002.

Chia, M. *Taoist Secrets of Love: Cultivating Male Sexual Energy*. Santa Fe, NM: Aurora Press, 1984.

Douglas, N. *Spiritual Sex: Secrets of Tantra from the Ice Age to the New Millennium.* New York: Pocket Books, 1997.

Sevely, J. L. *Eve's Secrets: A New Theory of Female Sexuality.* New York: Random House, 1987.

Stifter, K. *Die Dritte Dimension Der Lust—Das Geheimnis Der Weiblichen Ejakulation* [*The third dimension of lust: the secrets of female ejaculation.*] Frankfurt: Ullstein, 1988.

Strikes, T., and J. Orsi. *Song of the Deer: The Great Sundance Journey of the Soul.* Malibu, CA: Jaguar Books, 1999.

Stubbs, K. R. *Women of the Light: The New Sacred Prostitute.* Tucson, AZ: Secret Garden Publishing, 1997.

CHAPTER 4: EJACULATE WITHOUT AN ORGASM

Chopra, D. *Perfect Health.* New York: Random House, 1991.

Eichel, E. W. "Coital Orgasm Defined by the CAT Research." *Abstracts Book of the 13th World Congress on Sexuality and Human Rights.* Valencia, Spain, 1997.

Eichel, E. W., J. D. Eichel, and S. Kule. 1988. "The Technique of Coital Alignment and its Relation to Female Orgasmic Response and Simultaneous Orgasm." *Journal of Sex and Marital Therapy* 14:129–141.

Perry, J. D., and B. Whipple. 1981. "Pelvic Muscle Strength of Female Ejaculators: Evidence in Support of a New Theory of Orgasm." *Journal of Sex Research* 17:22–39.

Sivananda Yoga Center. *Sivananda Companion to Yoga.* New York: Simon and Schuster, 1983.

Sovatsky, S. *Passions of Innocence: Tantric Celibacy and the Mysteries of Eros.* Rochester, NY: Destiny Books, 1994.

Zaviacic, M., J. Jakubovsky, S. Polak, A. Zaviacicova, and I. K. Holoman. 1984. "Rhythmic Changes of Human Female Uroepithelial Squamous Cells During Menstrual Cycle." *International Urology and Nephrology* 16:301–309.

Zaviacic, M., I. K. Zaviacicova, and J. Molcan. 1988. "Female Urethral Expulsions Evoked by Local Digital Stimulation of the G-Spot: Differences in the Response Patterns." *Journal of Sex Research* 24:311–8.

CHAPTER 5: EJACULATE WITH AN ORGASM

Cameron, J. *The Artist's Way.* New York: Tarcher/Putnam, 1992.

Davis, E. *Women's Sexual Passages.* Alameda, CA.: Hunter House Publishers, 2000

Dodson, B. *Sex For One: The Joy of Selfloving.* Westminster, MD: Harmony Books, 1986. Reissued New York: Three Rivers Press, 1996.

Estes, C. P. *Women Who Run with the Wolves*. New York: Ballantine Books, 1992.

Goldberg, N. *Writing Down the Bones.* Boston, MA: Shambhala Publications, 1986.

Hines, T. 2001. "The G-Spot: A Modern Gynecological Myth." *American Journal of Obstetrics and Gynecology* 185:359–62.

Kinsey, A., et al. *Sexual Behavior in the Human Female.* Philadelphia, PA: W.B. Saunders, 1973.

Lessing, D. *The Golden Notebook*. Harmondsworth, U.K.: Penguin Books, 1964.

Masters, W., and V. Johnson. *Human Sexual Response.* Boston, MA: Little, Brown, 1966.

Odgen, G. *Women Who Love Sex.* New York: Pocket Books, 1994.

Roth, G. *The Wave.* New York: Bluehorse Films, 1997.

Singer, J., and I. Singer. "Types of Female Orgasm." In *Handbook of Sex Therapy,* edited by J. Lo Piccolo and L. Lo Piccolo. New York: Plenum Press, 1979, 175–86.

CHAPTER 6: EJACULATE WITH A PARTNER

Gray, J. *Mars and Venus on a Date*. New York: HarperCollins, 1992.

Stewart, J. *The Complete Manual of Sexual Positions.* Chatsworth, CA: Pacific Media Entertainment, 2002

Stubbs, K. R. *Kama Sutra of Sexual Positions*. Tucson, AZ: Secret Garden Publishing, 2001.

Sundahl, D. *How to Female Ejaculate for Couples: Share Your G-Spot.* Santa Fe, NM: Isis Media, 2002.

CHAPTER 7: MEN'S ROLE IN FEMALE EJACULATION

Anand, M. *The Art of Orgasm for Men.* Sebastapol, CA: Higher Love Video, 2000.

Chia, M. and D. Abrams. *The Multi-Orgasmic Man*. San Francisco, CA: Harper Collins, 1996.

Cote, M. *Be the Man of Her Fantasies!* Vancouver: Ishtara Seminars, 2001.

Gold, V. "Confessions of a Sexual Healer." Mill Valley, CA: unpublished manuscript, 2002.

Johnston, J. "Male Multiple Orgasm Step by Step," 4th ed. Ashland, OR: Jack Johnston Seminars, 2001 (audio tape).

Kramer, J. *Fire on the Mountain*. Oakland, CA: Joseph Kramer Productions, 1992 (video).

Muir, C., and C. Muir. *Tantra: The Art of Conscious Loving.* San Francisco, CA: Mercury House, 1989.

CHAPTER 8: HEAL YOUR G-SPOT

Anand, M. *The Art of Sexual Ecstasy.* New York: Tarcher/Putnam, 1989.

Anapol, D., and J. Painter. *Pelvic Heart Integration, Tape II.* San Rafael, CA: Sacred Space Institute, 2002.

Gold, V. "Confessions of a Sexual Healer." Mill Valley, CA: unpublished manuscript, 2003.

Ince, J. "Erotophobia" Vancouver: unpublished work, 2002.

Dodson, B. "Viva La Vulva: Women's Sex Organs Revealed." New York: Betty Dodson, 1998 (video).

Jwala. *Sacred Sex*. San Rafael, CA: Mandala Books, 1993.

Kramer, J., *Exploring the Land Down Under.* Oakland, CA: Joseph Kramer Productions, 1993 (video).

Kramer, J. *Fire on the Mountain*. Oakland, CA: Joseph Kramer Productions, 1992 (video).

Kramer, J. *Uranus: Self Anal Massage for Men.* Oakland, CA: Joseph Kramer Productions, 1996 (video).

Kramer, J., ed. *The Best of Vulva Massage*. Oakland, CA: Joseph Kramer Productions, 2002 (video).

Kramer, J., and A. Sprinkle. *Fire in the Valley: An Intimate Guide to Female Genital Massage*. Oakland, CA: Joseph Kramer Productions, 1999 (video).

Lowen, A. *Love and Orgasm.* New York: American Library, 1967.

Magdalena, I. 1997, "Celebrating the Body Electric for Women." *The Harvard Gay and Lesbian Review* IV, no. 3.

Muir, C., and C. Muir. *Freeing the Female Orgasm: Awakening the Goddess.* Maui, HI: Hawaiian Goddess Publishing, 1993.

Muir, C., and C. Muir. *Tantra: The Art of Conscious Loving*. San Francisco, CA: Mercury House, 1989.

Orloff, J. *Dr. Judith Orloff's Guide to Intuitive Healing: Five Steps to Physical, Emotional and Sexual Wellness.* New York: Random House, 2000.

Reich, W. *The Function of Orgasm,* translated by V. Carfagano. New York: Simon and Schuster, 1973.

Stubbs, K. R. *The Essential Tantra: A Modern Day Guide to Sacred Sex.* New York: Tarcher/Putnam, 1999.

Stubbs, K. R. *Tantric Massage Video.* Tucson, AZ: Secret Garden Publishing, 1994.

Sundahl, D. "Spiritual Access." In *Sex Tips and Tales,* edited by J. Baker. Alameda, CA: Hunter House, 2001.

Sundahl, D. *Tantric Journey to Female Orgasm: Awaken Your G-Spot.* Santa Fe, NM: Isis Media, 1998.

CHAPTER 9: CONNECTION TO SELF AND PARTNER

Anand, M. *The Art of Sexual Ecstasy.* New York: Tarcher/Putnam, 1989.

Douglas, N. *Spiritual Sex: Secrets of Tantra from the Ice Age to the New Millennium.* New York: Pocket Books, 1997.

Muir, C., and C. Muir. *Female Sexual Ecstasy: Awakening the Goddess.* Maui, HI: Source Tantra School of Yoga, 1996.

Steinberg, D. *The Erotic Impulse: Honoring the Sensual Self.* New York: Tarcher/Perigee, 1992.

Stubbs, K. R. *The Essential Tantra: A Modern Day Guide to Sacred Sex.* New York: Tarcher/Putnam, 1999.

Wilson, R. A. *Coincidence.* Scottsdale, AZ: New Falcon, 1991.

Resources

◆

ⓖ G-Spot Toys and Information Sexuality Shops ⓖ

Clean, well-lighted places for women and men to shop for sex toys and erotic and sex education books and videos, and attend workshops on many aspects of sexuality.

Good Vibrations   www.goodvibes.com
    1210 Valencia St.   (800) 289-8423
    San Francisco CA

    2504 San Pablo Blvd.   (800) 289-8423
    Berkeley CA

Eve's Garden   www.evesgarden.com
    119 W. 57th St.   (800) 848-3837
    New York NY

Toys in Babeland   www.babeland.com
    707 E. Pike St.   (800) 658-9119
    Seattle WA

    94 Rivington St.   (800) 658-9119
    New York NY

Grand Opening!   www.grandopening.com
    318 Harvard St., #32 Arcade Bldg.   (877) 731-2626
    Boston MA

    8442 Santa Monica Blvd.   (323) 848-6970
    West Hollywood CA 90060   mail order: (877) 731-2626

The Love Boutique
  18637 Ventura Blvd.   (818) 342-2400
  Tarzana CA

  2924 Wilshire Blvd.   (310) 453-3459
  Santa Monica CA 90403

Come As You Are   www.comeasyouare.com
  701 Queen's St. W.   (877) 858-3160
  Toronto Ontario
  Canada

Good For Her   www.goodforher.com
  175 Harbord St.   (877) 588-0900
  Toronto Ontario
  Canada

☉ Recommended G-Spot Sex Toys ☽
and Ejaculation Products

The following are innovative sex toys developed by female sex educators specifically for the G-spot. They were recommended in this book and are not readily available at the sexuality shops listed above.

The Deluxe Crystal Wand, Taylor Lamborne, www.lovenectar.com

The Love Handle, limited edition, Dr. Annie Sprinkle,
www.gatesofheck.com/annie

Ejaculation Bowls, limited edition, Deborah Sundahl, www.isismedia.org

Sheet Savers, Karen Fowler, www.getinthemood.com,
(866) LUV-LINR (588-5467)

☉ Sexuality Mail-Order Catalogs ☽
and Internet Shopping

The reputable stores listed above and a few other selected companies offer many of the items listed in this resource section or recommended in this book by mail, via the Internet, or by telephone.

www.asstroknots.com

www.babeland.com   (800) 658-9119

www.evesgarden.com   (800) 848-3837

www.goodvibes.com   (800) 289-8423

www.grandopening.com   (877) 731-2626

www.loveandintimacy.com

www.lovenectar.com

www.pleasurespot.com.au

www.secretgardenpublishing.com

www.tantra.com   (800) 982-6872

www.xandria.com

⊚ Books ⊚

For further information on female ejaculation, the G-spot, and sacred sexuality, I highly recommend these books.

Female Ejaculation and the G-Spot

Federation of Feminist Women's Health Care Centers. *A New View of a Woman's Body*, 2nd ed. Illustrated by Suzann Gage. Los Angeles, CA: Feminist Health Press, 1991.

Ladas, A., B. Whipple, and J. Perry. *The G-Spot and Other Discoveries about Human Sexuality.* New York: Holt, Rinehart and Winston, 1982; New York: Dell, 1983.

Sevely, J. L. *Eve's Secrets: A New Theory of Female Sexuality.* New York: Random House, 1987.

Stewart, J. *The Complete Manual of Sexual Positions*. Chatsworth, CA: Pacific Media Entertainment, 2002

Stewart, J. *Sexual Secrets: The Lover's Guide to Sexual Ecstasy*. Chatsworth, CA: Pacific Media Entertainment, 2001

Stifter, K. *Die Dritte Dimension Der Lust—Das Geheimnis Der Weiblichen Ejakulation* [*The Third Dimension of Lust: The Secrets of Female Ejaculation*.] Frankfurt: Ullstein, 1988.

Stubbs, K. R., with L. Saulnier. *Erotic Massage*. New York: J. P. Tarcher, 1999.

Stubbs, K. R., with L. Saulnier. *Erotic Passions*, revised and expanded edition. New York: J. P. Tarcher, 2000.

Winks, C. *The Good Vibrations Guide: The G-Spot*. Berkeley, CA: Down There Press, 1998.

Zaviacic, M. *The Human Female Prostate: From Vestigial Skene's Paraurethral Glands and Ducts to Woman's Functional Prostate*. Bratislava: Slovak Academic Press, 1999.

Sexual Healing and Spiritual Sex

Anand, M. *The Art of Sexual Ecstasy*. New York: Tarcher/Putnam, 1989.

Chia, M. *Healing Love Through the Tao: Cultivating Female Sexual Energy*. Lodi, NJ: Healing Tao, 1991.

Douglas, N. *Spiritual Sex: Secrets of Tantra from the Ice Age to the New Millennium*. New York: Pocket Books, 1997.

Jwala. *Sacred Sex*. San Rafael, CA: Mandala Books, 1993.

Orloff, J. *Intuitive Healing: Five Steps to Developing Intuition*. Carlsbad, CA: Hay House, 2002.

Stubbs, K. R. *The Essential Tantra: A Modern Day Guide to Sacred Sex*. New York: Tarcher/Putnam, 1999.

☉ Audiotapes and Audio CDs ☉

Female Ejaculation and the G-Spot

"How to Female Ejaculate: Step by Step Practice Guide" by Deborah Sundahl, www.isismedia.org

Sexual Healing and Spiritual Sex

"The Art of Everyday Ecstasy" by Deepak Chopra and Margo Anand, www.tantra.com

☉ Videos/DVDs ☉

Below are cutting-edge videos and DVDs on sex education, the G-spot, female ejaculation, and sacred sex, produced by pioneering sex educators.

Female Ejaculation

Lane, D., and House O' Chicks. *The Magic of Female Ejaculation*. San Francisco, CA: House O'Chicks, 1992.

Perry, M. *The Amazing G-Spot and Female Ejaculation*. Encino, CA: Access International, 1999.

Sundahl, D. *How to Female Ejaculate: Find Your G-Spot with Deborah Sundahl*. Santa Fe, NM: Isis Media, 2002.

Sundahl, D. *How to Female Ejaculate for Couples: Share Your G-Spot*. Santa Fe, NM: Isis Media, 2003.

Sundahl, D. *Tantric Journey to Female Orgasm: Awaken Your G-Spot.* Santa Fe, NM: Isis Media, 1998.

G-Spot

Anand, M. *The Art of Orgasm for Women*. Sebastapol, CA: Higher Love Video, 2000.

Kramer, J., and A. Sprinkle. *Fire in the Valley: An Intimate Guide to Female Genital Massage*. Oakland, CA: Joseph Kramer Productions, 1999.

Muir, C., and C. Muir. *Secrets of Female Sexual Ecstasy.* Kahului, HI: Charles and Caroline Muir Source School of Tantra, 1996.

Sprinkle, A., and M. Beatty. *Sluts and Goddesses*. Oakland, CA: Joseph Kramer Productions, 1992.

Sprinkle, A., and D. Lane. *Masturbation Memoirs*. San Francisco, CA: House O' Chicks, 1994.

Stewart, J. *The Complete Manual of Sexual Positions*. Chatsworth, CA: Pacific Media Entertainment, 1995.

Stewart, J. *The Lovers Guide to Sexual Ecstasy*. Chatsworth, CA: Pacific Media Entertainment, 1992.

Stubbs, K. R. *Tantric Massage Video*. Tucson, AZ: Secret Garden Publishing, 1994.

Sacred Sexuality

Painter, J. *Pelvic Heart Integration: Part 2,* San Rafael: Deborah Anapol, 2002

Expand Her Orgasm Tonight: A Pleasurable Guide for Partners. Chatsworth, CA: Pacific Media Entertainment, 1999.

⊚ Female Ejaculation Websites ⊚

www.drGSpot.net (Dr. John Perry's website)
This site provides the best educational information on female ejaculation and the G-spot available on the Internet.

TheGSpot@yahoogroups.com (to subscribe, send an email with the words "I wish to subscribe" to this email address)

www.isismedia.org

www.DoctorG.com

www.houseochicks.com

☺ Female Ejaculation Workshops ☺

The individuals listed below are established female-ejaculation sex educators.

Online Workshops

Deborah Sundahl, www.isismedia.org

In-Person Workshops

Shannon Bell, Ph.D., shanbell@yorku.ca (Toronto, Canada)

Kirn Airs, Grand Opening!, www.grandopening.com (Brookline/Boston, MA)

Deborah Sundahl, Isis Media, www.isismedia.org (Midwest/Southwest USA)

Dori Lane, House O'Chicks, www.houseochicks.com (San Francisco, CA)

☺ G-Spot Awakening Workshops ☺

Experienced and inspired sacred sex educators who have included G-spot (sacred spot) and female ejaculation information in their workshops.

Taylor Lamborne, Nectar Products www.lovenectar.com (San Diego, CA)

Margo Anand, Skydancing Institute, www.margoanand.com

Charles and Caroline Muir, Source Tantra, www.sourcetantra.com

Jwala, Tantric Priestess, www.tantra.com/jwala

Ina Laughing Winds, Sacred Living International, www.spiritualsexuality.com (Phoenix, AZ)

Corynna Clarke, Temple of the Goddess, www.goddesstemple.com

Deborah Anapol, Sacred Space Institute, www.lovewithoutlimits.com

Isa Magdelena, women's sexuality educator, xtasia@toasnet.com

ⓖ Recommended Products for ⓔ
PC-Muscles Fitness

The list below includes the exercise products and list of clinics recommended in this book for pelvic-muscle fitness.

The Fria Biofeedback Perineometer (www.drGSpot.net)

The Crystal Onyx Vaginal Weight Lifting Egg (www.lovenectar.com)

Goddess Vaginal Strengthening Egg (www.tantra.com)

List of perineometer clinics (www.drGSpot.net)

Herbal lubricant (www.isismedia.org)

ⓖ Books for Breathing Techniques ⓔ

Located within the text of these two excellent books are breathing techniques that produce noticeable relaxation for awakening the G-spot and male ejaculation control.

Chopra, D. *Perfect Health: The Complete Mind-Body Guide.* New York: Three Rivers Press, 2001

Vishnu-Devananda, S. *The Sivananda Companion to Yoga: A Complete Guide to the Physical Postures, Breathing* Exercises, Diet, Relaxation, and Meditation Techniques of Yoga. New York: Simon & Schuster, 2000

ⓖ For Men: More Pleasure, Less Control ⓔ

Useful information on this new and important topic for men can be found in the listings below.

Books

Chang, S. T. *The Tao of Sexology: The Book of Infinite Wisdom.* San Francisco, CA: Tao Publishing, 1986

Chia, M. and D. Abrams. *The Multi-Orgasmic Man.* San Francisco, CA: HarperCollins, 1996.

Chia, M. *Taoist Secrets of Love: Cultivating Male Sexual Energy.* Santa Fe, NM: Aurora Press, 1984.

Videos

Anand, M. *The Art of Orgasm for Men.* Petaluma, CA: Higher Love Video, 2000. <www.tantra.com>

Kramer, J. *Evolutionary Masturbation: An Intimate Guide to the Male Orgasm.* Oakland, CA: Joseph Kramer, 1998. <www.eroticmassage.com>

"Lover's Guide to Ejaculation Control: Master Your Pleasure." Pacific Media Entertainment. <www.loveandintimacy.com>

Audiotapes and Audio CDs

Ishtara. "Sexercise Training: Total Ejaculation Control for Men." San Rafael, CA: Ishtara, 1995. <www.tantra.com>

Johnston, J. "Male Multiple Orgasms Step by Step!" Ashland, OR: Jack Johnston Seminars, 2001. <www.multlples.com>

Internet Forums

www.malemultipleorgasms.com

⊙ Sexual Healing Schools and Instructors ⊚

These sexual healing schools offer classes to instructors and individuals across the United States and in Australia and Canada, as well as online.

In Person

Body Electric School, Ken Oakley, Oakland, CA; Collin Brown and Selah Martha, Port Townsend, WA <www.bodyelectric.org>

Daka/Dakini School, Dr. Corynna Clarke. <www.goddesstemple.com>

Erosha Institute, John Ince, Vancouver, Canada. <www.erosha.com>

Online

New School of Erotic Touch, Joseph Kramer. <www.eroticmassage.com>

Videos for Self-Instruction

"Best of Vulva Massage." Joseph Kramer, Joseph Kramer Productions

"Tantric Journey to Female Orgasm: Awaken Your G-Spot." Deborah Sundahl, Isis Media

"Tantric Massage Video I and II." Kenneth Ray Stubbs, Secret Garden Publishing

Index

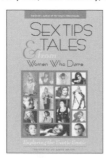
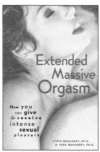

THE POCKET BOOK OF SENSATIONAL ORGASMS *by* Richard Craze

This is a unique look at how partners can intensify, extend, and enhance orgasms. Using techniques such as "The Tail of the Ostrich" and the "Two-Handed Twist," partners can release inhibitions and share erotic adventures. The book also explains the difference between male and female orgasms; types of orgasms: vaginal, clitoral, G-spot, anal, multiple, mutual, and oral; and how to magnify sexual satisfaction with seduction and foreplay.

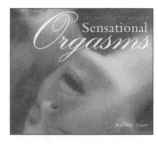

96 pages ... 64 color photos ... Paperback $11.95

SIMULTANEOUS ORGASM and Other Joys of Sexual Intimacy *by* Michael Riskin, Ph.D., & Anita Banker-Riskin, M.A.

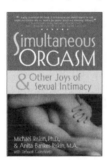

Based on techniques developed at the Human Sexuality Institute, this guide shows couples how they can achieve the special, intimate experience of simultaneous orgasm. The book gives specific techniques and step-by-step instructions that help individuals achieve orgasm separately, and then simultaneously. Exercises include practical advice for relaxing and feeling comfortable with yourself and your partner. A separate section explains the purpose of the exercise and offers insights about how it can positively affect your relationship.

240 pages ... 9 b/w photos ... Paperback $14.95 ... Hardcover $24.95

SEXUAL PLEASURE: Reaching New Heights of Sexual Arousal and Intimacy *by* Barbara Keesling

This book is for anyone who wants to make love without anxiety or pressure, which starts with learning to enjoy touching and being touched. It shows how to focus on your desire, which puts you in touch with your body.

Sexual Pleasure introduces readers to unique **sensate focus** exercises, to be done alone and with a partner, to increase sensual awareness. The exercises are independent of sexual orientation and can be used by those who have physical limitations, those who are learning about sexuality—anyone interested in better sex.

224 pages ... 14 b/w photos ... Paperback $14.95

To order or for our FREE catalog or call (800) 266-5592

ORDER FORM

NAME

ADDRESS

CITY/STATE   ZIP/POSTCODE

PHONE   COUNTRY (outside of U.S.)

TITLE	QTY	PRICE	TOTAL
Female Ejaculation & the G-Spot (paper)		@ $ 15.95	
Sex Tips and Tales from Women... (paper)		@ $ 13.95	

Prices subject to change without notice

Please list other titles below:

		@ $	
		@ $	
		@ $	
		@ $	
		@ $	
		@ $	
		@ $	

Check here to receive our book catalog ☐   FREE

Shipping Costs

By Priority Mail: first book $4.50, each additional book $1.00
By UPS and to Canada: first book $5.50, each additional book $1.50
For rush orders and other countries call us at (510) 865-5282

TOTAL _____
Less discount @_____% (_____)
TOTAL COST OF BOOKS _____
Calif. residents add sales tax _____
Shipping & handling _____
TOTAL ENCLOSED _____

Please pay in U.S. funds only

☐ Check   ☐ Visa   ☐ MasterCard   ☐ Discover

Card #_____ Exp. date_____

Signature_____

Complete and mail to:
Hunter House Inc., Publishers
PO Box 2914, Alameda CA 94501-0914
Website: www.hunterhouse.com
Orders: (800) 266-5592 or email: ordering@hunterhouse.com
Phone (510) 865-5282   Fax (510) 865-4295

FEJ 3/2003